M000301878

UNIPAC Five: *Caring for the Terminally Ill—Communication and the Physician's Role on the Interdisciplinary Team*

Second Edition

Porter Storey, MD, FACP, FAAHPM
Associate Professor of Medicine
Section of Geriatrics
Baylor College of Medicine

Consultant in the Department of Symptom Control and Palliative Care
University of Texas MD Anderson Cancer Center

Medical Director
Palliative Care Services
St. Luke's Episcopal Hospital
Houston, Texas

Carol F. Knight, EdM
Knight Consultants
Austin, Texas

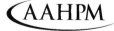

American Academy of Hospice and Palliative Medicine

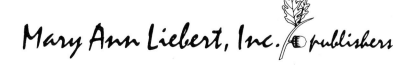

The information presented and opinions expressed herein are those of the authors and do not necessarily represent the views of the sponsor or its parent agencies, the National Institutes of Health, the United States Public Health Service, the reviewers, or a consensus of the members of the American Academy of Hospice and Palliative Medicine. Any recommendations made by the authors must be weighed against the physician's own clinical judgment, based on but not limited to such factors as the patient's condition, benefits versus risks of suggested treatment, and comparison with recommendations of pharmaceutical compendia and other authorities.

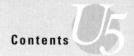

Contents

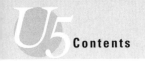

Contents

AAHPM

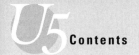

Contents

Tables

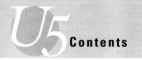

Contents

The authors and the American Academy of Hospice and Palliative Medicine (AAHPM) are deeply grateful to the following reviewers for their participation in the development of this component of the Academy's self-study curriculum, *Hospice/Palliative Care Training for Physicians: UNIPACs*. The reviewers' extensive comments and thoughtful suggestions greatly improved its contents. We want to express special gratitude to the following physicians who also recruited field testers and coordinated local testing of the UNIPAC: Gerald Holman, MD, Eli Perencevich, DO, and Julia Smith, MD. Finally our special thanks to all the practicing physicians, fellows, residents, and medical students who participated in evaluating this component of the Academy's physician training curriculum.

John W. Finn, MD
Medical Director
Hospice of Michigan
Southfield, Michigan

Walter B. Forman, MD
Professor of Medicine and Geriatrics
University of New Mexico School of
    Medicine
Albuquerque, New Mexico

Rev. Milton W. Hay, DMin
Former Spiritual Caregiver Section Leader
National Council of Hospice Professionals
National Hospice Organization
Pacific Grove, California

Michael E. Frederich, MD
Clinical Instructor
Department of Family and Preventive
    Medicine
School of Medicine
Medical Director, Palliative Home Healthcare
San Diego Hospice
San Diego, California

Barbara M. Henley, LMSW, ACP
Special Assistant to the Dean
University of Houston
Graduate School of Social Work
Houston, Texas

Gerald H. Holman, MD
Founding Chairman, Board of Trustees
American Board of Hospice and Palliative
    Medicine
Amarillo, Texas

Rev. Charles Meyer, MDiv, MS
Former Vice-President
St. David's Hospital
Austin, Texas

Terry C. Muck, PhD
Professor of Comparative Religion
Austin Presbyterian Theological Seminary
Austin, Texas

Eli N. Perencevich, DO
Clinical Assistant Professor of Medicine
Ohio State University
Medical Director
Hospice of Columbus
Columbus, Ohio

Charles G. Sasser, MD
Medical Director
Mercy Hospice of Horry County
Conway, South Carolina

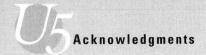

Acknowledgments

Julia L. Smith, MD
Division Chief, Oncology/Hematology
Genesee Hospital
Associate Professor, Oncology in Medicine
University of Rochester
Medical Director, Hospice of Rochester
Rochester, New York

Bradley Stuart, MD
Medical Director
VNA and Hospice of Northern California
Santa Rosa, California

Academy's Physician Training Programs

The Academy recognizes the need for physician education on palliative medicine at the end of life and has designed its physician training programs to meet its own education goals, as well as those of the National Cancer Institute. The training programs include the following:

Hospice/Palliative Medicine: Self-Study Program for Physicians

The Academy's self-study program consists of a series of monographs, or UNIPACs, each of which follows the recommended format for self-instructional learning, including behavioral objectives, a pretest, reading material, clinical situations for demonstrating knowledge application, a posttest, and references. The self-study program was made possible with federal funds from the National Cancer Institute's Cancer Education Grant Program, Grant CA66771. The following UNIPACs are approved for CME credit:

- *UNIPAC One: The Hospice/Palliative Medicine Approach to End-of-Life Care*
- *UNIPAC Two: Alleviating Psychological and Spiritual Pain in the Terminally Ill*
- *UNIPAC Three: Assessment and Treatment of Pain in the Terminally Ill*
- *UNIPAC Four: Management of Selected Non-pain Symptoms in the Terminally Ill*
- *UNIPAC Five: Caring for the Terminally Ill—Communication and the Physician's Role on the Interdisciplinary Team*
- *UNIPAC Six: Ethical and Legal Decision Making When Caring for the Terminally Ill*
- *UNIPAC Seven: The Hospice/Palliative Medicine Approach to Caring for Patients with AIDS*
- *UNIPAC Eight: The Hospice/Palliative Medicine Approach to Caring for Pediatric Patients*

Although the UNIPACs may be used when studying for the American Board of Hospice and Palliative Medicine's written examination for certification, they were not developed for that purpose. The Academy recommends that candidates for the examination review selected references listed at the end of each UNIPAC and other materials relevant to the examination.

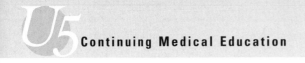

Pocket Guide to Hospice/Palliative Medicine

The *Pocket Guide to Hospice/Palliative Medicine* is a concise, clinically oriented reference for residents and practicing physicians. It consists primarily of tables and assessment tools from the Academy's self study program, *Hospice/Palliative Medicine: A Self-Study Program for Physicians.* Development of the Pocket Guide was made possible with federal funds from the National Cancer Institute's Cancer Education Grant Program, Grant CA66771.

Hospice and Palliative Medicine: Core Curriculum and Review Syllabus

The Academy's core curriculum and review syllabus, *Hospice and Palliative Medicine: Core Curriculum and Review Syllabus,* presents the core elements of hospice and palliative medicine identified by the Institute of Medicine as essential for effective end-of-life care. The document consists of a series of modules, each of which includes a brief narrative summary of a specific topic, objectives, and references. The curriculum was the first one in the United States developed primarily by palliative medicine physicians.

Primer of Palliative Care

The *Primer of Palliative Care* is a brief introduction to palliative care that covers the history of hospice, the basic elements of hospice and palliative care, pain and symptom management techniques, and alleviation of psychological, social, and spiritual distress. The Primer includes an annotated bibliography.

For more information on the Academy's physician training programs, call the AAHPM at (847) 375-4712 or fax (847) 375-6312.

Continuing Medical Education

Purpose

A UNIPAC is a packet of information formatted as a self-study program. It includes learning objectives, a pretest, reading material, clinical situations for demonstrating knowledge application, a posttest, and references. This self-study program is intended for physicians and physicians-in-training. It is designed to increase competence in palliative medical interventions for improving a patient's quality of life, particularly as death approaches. Specific, practical information is presented to help physicians assess and manage selected problems. After reading the UNIPAC, physicians are encouraged to seek additional training in hospice/palliative medicine.

Learning Objectives

Upon completion of this continuing medical education program, a physician should be better able to:

- Use effective strategies when communicating with patients, families, and other healthcare professionals.

- Use effective techniques when communicating bad news.

- Use knowledge of family systems theory and counseling techniques to facilitate family conferences.

- Use knowledge of the roles and functions of team members to interact more effectively as a team member.

- Use conflict-resolution skills to promote effective team work.

- Use knowledge of basic issues to guide decisions about respecting confidentiality

- Use effective techniques to manage the stress associated with caring for terminally ill patients.

Recommended Procedure

To receive maximum benefit from this UNIPAC, the following procedure is recommended:

- Complete the pretest before reading the UNIPAC.

- Review the learning objectives.

- Study each section and the clinical situations.

- Review the correct responses to the pretest.

- Complete the posttest by marking your answers on the answer sheet.

Accreditation Statement

The American Academy of Hospice and Palliative Medicine (AAHPM) is accredited by the Accreditation Council for Continuing Medical Education (ACCME) to provide continuing medical education for physicians.

CAAHPM

The AAHPM designates this continuing medical education activity for a maximum of six (6) hours in Category 1 towards the AMA Physician's Recognition Award.

Physicians are eligible to receive credit by completing and returning the evaluation form and the posttest answer sheet to the AAHPM. The Academy will keep a record of AMA/PRA Category 1 credit hours and the record will be provided on request; however, physicians are responsible for reporting their own Category 1 CME credits when applying for the AMA/PRA or for other certificates or credentials. Each physician should claim only those hours of credit that he or she actually spent in the activity.

Disclosure

All faculty are required to disclose to program participants any relationship, including financial interest or affiliation(s), with a commercial company, as well as discussion of unlabeled uses. The program authors have disclosed information on sources of funding for research, consulting agreements, offices in professional associations, financial interests, and stock ownership.

Porter Storey, MD, once served on the speakers' bureau for Purdue Pharmaceuticals and has received research support from the National Cancer Institute. **Carol F. Knight, EdM,** has received research support from the National Cancer Institute.

Review and Revision

Reviewed and re-approved by the American Academy of Hospice and Palliative Medicine's Publications and CME Committees: May 2002.

Term of Offering

The release date for the second edition of this UNIPAC is April, 2003, and the expiration date is December 31, 2006. Final date to request credit is December 31, 2006.

Posttest Pass Rate

The posttest pass rate is 75%.

Additional Information

Additional information is available from the American Academy of Hospice and Palliative Medicine, where staff can direct you to physicians specializing in end-of-life care.

This self-study program was supported in part by federal funds from the National Cancer Institute's Cancer Education Grant Program, Grant CA66771.

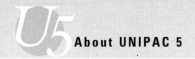

Evaluation Form

Use this evaluation form to rate the UNIPAC that you have completed according to the five criteria listed and then mail or fax the form to the Academy at the address below. To receive CME credit, follow the same procedure.

Currency of information	__Excellent	__Good	__Fair	__Poor
Clarity of presentation	__Excellent	__Good	__Fair	__Poor
Content of material	__Excellent	__Good	__Fair	__Poor
Effectiveness of teaching method	__Excellent	__Good	__Fair	__Poor
Relevance to my practice	__Excellent	__Good	__Fair	__Poor

Suggestions for improving the enduring material:

Mail or fax to:
American Academy of Hospice and Palliative Medicine
4700 W. Lake Avenue
Glenview, Illinois 60025-1485
Phone: 847/375-4761
Fax: 847/375-4777

Pretest

Before proceeding, complete the following multiple-choice items. The correct responses are included at the end of the UNIPAC.

1. **Which of the following statements is true?**

   A. Most patients believe that information about their diagnosis and prognosis benefits them, even when the news is bad.

   B. The manner in which bad news about a diagnosis is communicated is less important than the inclusion of complete descriptions of all test results.

   C. Experienced, skilled physicians can easily determine how much information patients want about diagnosis and prognosis.

   D. When a physician's nonverbal cues contradict a verbal message, patients are much more likely to believe the physician's verbal statements.

2. **A patient's reluctance to discuss diagnosis and prognosis is likely to result from all the following *except* which one?**

   A. A need to periodically deny the existence of a life-threatening condition

   B. The widespread belief among patients that information about diagnosis and prognosis will do them harm

   C. The desire to protect themselves, their family members, and their physicians from the distressing emotions that often accompany discussions of poor prognosis

   D. Subtle, nonverbal cues from the physician indicating that such discussions are unwelcome

3. **All the following statements are true *except* which one?**

   A. Honest communication increases a patient's and family's sense of control and self-worth.

   B. For terminally ill patients, a sense of being heard may be the most effective healing agent.

   C. Because unrelieved symptoms and stress interfere with a patient's ability to hear and retain information, physicians should first focus on alleviating distressing symptoms, establishing a therapeutic relationship, and repeating information as often as needed.

   D. Poor communication skills may interfere with a physician's ability to perform an adequate history, but they have little impact on the patient's overall sense of suffering.

AAHPM

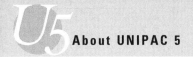

4. **All the following statements are true *except* which one?**

   A. There is little correlation between the likelihood of a medical malpractice suit and a physician's ability to communicate effectively.

   B. A physician's ability to communicate effectively with patients is affected by the physician's own intrapersonal communication.

   C. Effective communication with patients during the history-taking process contributes more information about diagnosis than laboratory tests.

   D. Therapeutic communication is important, even when interacting with comatose patients.

5. **All the following statements are true *except* which one?**

   A. A patient's most basic needs are the need to know and understand the diagnosis and prognosis and the need to feel known and understood by the physician.

   B. When physicians interact with patients, just the act of sitting down increases patient satisfaction.

   C. A light-hearted approach to terminal illness increases patient satisfaction.

   D. Patient satisfaction depends more on the perception of a physician's emotional support and adequate sharing of information than on the amount of time that the physician actually spends with patients.

6. **Which of the following statements about communication is correct?**

   A. To ensure effective communication with patients, most physicians can easily switch from medical language to everyday language.

   B. When dying patients have limited English language skills, physicians can rely on the patient's friends and/or family members to provide reliable interpretation.

   C. When physicians engage in meaningful communication and try to understand a patient's point of view, their own long-held beliefs may be challenged by the patient's beliefs and experiences.

   D. Most physicians, nurses, and patients understand commonly used medical and psychological terms.

7. **In most situations, which of the following nonverbal behaviors is *least likely* to communicate empathy?**

   A. Sitting down so that the physician's eyes are slightly lower than the patient's.

   B. Sitting very close to the patient, about 12 to 18 inches

C. Sitting about 20 to 36 inches from the patient

D. Sitting in a relaxed position and leaning toward the patient

8. **All the following statements about communication techniques, such as listening, acknowledging, clarifying, reassuring, and validating, are true *except* which one?**

A. They can serve as powerful treatment interventions.

B. They can influence a patient's expectations.

C. They can affect the patient's emotional and physical well-being.

D. They encourage patients to focus exclusively on physical symptoms.

9. **Which of the following statements is correct?**

A. Physicians tend to interrupt their patients within the first 18 seconds of an interview.

B. Minimal leads such as "Uh-huh," "Umm," and "Ah" are ineffective listening techniques.

C. Confrontation is an inappropriate technique in palliative care settings.

D. The following is an example of repetition: "What is going on when you are not feeling good?"

10. **All the following statements about empathy are true *except* which one?**

A. Empathy refers to the ability to identify a patient's emotions.

B. Empathy refers to the ability to hear the unspoken questions and messages that lie underneath a patient's words.

C. Empathic response requires physical contact such as a hug or a pat on the back.

D. Empathy refers to the ability to recognize when listening is a more appropriate intervention than ordering additional medications or procedures.

11. **All the following statements are true *except* which one?**

A. To help terminally ill patients regain a sense of perspective, physicians should tell jokes and try to be funny.

B. Patients sometimes use humor as a powerful intervention for coping with loss.

C. Humor requires the ability to step back from a situation and recognize its paradoxical qualities.

D. Sensitivity and intuition are critical when using humor in the palliative care setting.

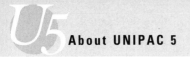

12. When physicians communicate bad news, patients prefer all the following *except* which one?

    A. Direct, empathic communication that includes information about diagnosis

    B. High levels of sustained optimism and continued emphasis on the positive aspects of the situation

    C. Information about prognosis and how it is likely to affect their plans for the future

    D. Inclusion of a family member or friend when bad news is shared

13. When sharing bad news, which of the following statements is correct?

    A. Avoid statements or inquiries that are likely to elicit painful emotions on the part of the patient or family.

    B. Use medical vocabulary so that patients and families can learn to speak intelligently about the patient's condition.

    C. First give a brief, rapid summary of the patient's diagnosis and prognosis; then go back over the information more slowly.

    D. When patients no longer appear to be listening, bring the interview to a close and reschedule a follow-up after patients and families have had time to assimilate the news.

14. When patients respond emotionally to bad news, which of the following statements is true?

    A. As soon as patients or family members start to cry, hand them a facial tissue.

    B. When patients respond with anger, the most important first step is to correct factual misconceptions.

    C. After emotions have cooled, trying to use a problem-solving approach will escalate the patient's anger.

    D. Anger is usually based on displaced fear and/or feelings of being ignored and devalued.

15. All the following statements about discussing prognosis are true *except* which one?

    A. Patients rarely want much information about prognosis.

    B. A precise estimate of life expectancy may become a fixed sentence in the patient's mind.

C. When patients request information about prognosis, physicians should provide estimates that are as accurate as possible.

D. Physicians should encourage patients to complete the developmental tasks of the dying.

16. **All the following statements about sharing bad news are true *except* which one?**

A. Communication should be an ongoing event, and the pace should be determined by the patient's personality and desire to know more.

B. Patients are more interested in diagnosis and treatment plans than in the illness's likely impact on themselves and their family members.

C. Physicians and nurses consistently underestimate the type and amount of information that patients want to know.

D. Most patients know that they are dying, so avoiding discussion of their prognosis is likely to increase their sense of isolation.

17. **When sharing bad news, which of the following statements is true?**

A. Physicians should wear white coats to emphasize their professional knowledge and authority.

B. Televisions and radios should be left on to provide welcome distractions from the bad news.

C. Physicians should provide reassurance by emphasizing that "everything is going to be fine."

D. Physicians should always sit down when sharing bad news.

18. **All the following statements about sharing bad news are true *except* which one?**

A. Use simple, everyday language (i.e., no medical jargon or euphemisms).

B. Fire "warning shots" to indicate that the situation is worse than expected, e.g., "I'm afraid your symptoms indicate that the illness is taking a turn for the worse."

C. The most important factor is determining precisely how much information a referring physician has shared with the patient about diagnosis and prognosis.

D. Repeat information as often as needed.

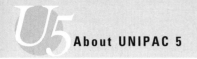

19. **When terminally ill patients first ask if they are dying, which of the following is most likely to be an appropriate response?**

   A. There is no need to talk about dying now. I'll let you know when the time comes to worry.

   B. It's hard to say; everyone is terminal. We're all dying.

   C. Yes. You probably have no more than _____ (fill in the correct number of days, weeks, or months) left to live.

   D. Based on the medical evidence, your situation does look very serious. What are some of your main concerns about dying?

20. **When terminally ill patients ask for more information about how much time they have left to live, which of the following is the most appropriate response?**

   A. I would guess about _____ (fill in a specific number of days, weeks, or months).

   B. There is really no point in trying to guess; everyone is different.

   C. There is always a lot of uncertainty when estimating length of life because people generally live longer or shorter than an average. Based on the medical indications and your situation, you are likely to live about _____ (fill in a range of estimated number of days, weeks, months, i.e. several weeks and maybe as much as a few months).

   D. I think such information would depress you and destroy all of your hope, so I prefer not to talk about it.

21. **After sharing bad news about diagnosis and prognosis, which of the following is the *least* appropriate role for a physician?**

   A. Help patients and families identify specific problems and distinguish those that are fixable from those that are not.

   B. Leave patients and families alone so that they can devise their own situation-specific solutions for coping.

   C. Help patients and families identify successful coping strategies and past and current sources of support.

   D. Remind patients and family members that the entire team will be available to answers questions, provide support, and help to resolve problems.

22. **Which of the following statements is correct?**

   A. Members of enmeshed families rarely experience significant grief-related problems because the family system's beliefs encourage individuals to develop identities apart from the family.

B. Functional enmeshment is particularly inappropriate when families are coping with a patient's terminal illness.

C. Members of open family systems rarely experience significant stress during a patient's terminal illness.

D. Members of open family systems are more likely to view change as inevitable and to use direct communication when talking about problems.

23. **A family system's response to terminal illness is likely to be affected by which of the following?**

A. The patient's roles in the family

B. The family system's rules regarding communication and interaction with the outside world

C. The ability of remaining family members to perform essential tasks

D. All the above

24. **When physicians participate in family conferences, which of the following behaviors is *least* appropriate?**

A. Exhibiting primary loyalty to the patient

B. Correcting misconceptions about diagnosis and treatments

C. Acknowledging the patient's and family's fears, grief, and guilt

D. Helping patients and families to identify strengths and set realistic short-term goals

25. **Which of the following statements about effective negotiation is correct?**

A. It clarifies the participants' views.

B. It focuses primarily on long-term goals.

C. It encourages rapid identification of a solution.

D. It discourages emphasis on each participant's dignity and self-esteem.

26. **Which of the following statements about family conferences is correct?**

A. Effective physicians are able to resolve the family's long-standing problems.

B. When counseling with patients and families, effective physicians involve other team members, such as a hospice/palliative care nurse, social worker, or chaplain.

C. Effective physicians can control the outcome of family conferences.

D. Physicians are responsible for the choices made by patients and family members.

(AAHPM

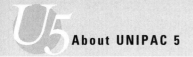

27. **All the following statements about denial are true *except* which one?**

    A. Denial is a commonly used unconscious response for coping with the implications of a terminal illness; it usually waxes and wanes throughout the course of the terminal illness.

    B. Whenever possible, physicians and other healthcare professionals should break down a patient's denial so that reality can be confronted more effectively.

    C. A family's insistence on withholding information from the patient is likely to result from the family members' own death-related fears.

    D. Instead of acquiescing with a family's demand to withhold information, physicians should help family members to explore their concerns, normalize their fears, and provide education.

28. **Which of the following statements about confidentiality is correct?**

    A. Team members are required to share all patient–family information with other members of the team.

    B. Confidentiality is breached when a team member shares confidential information without the patient's permission.

    C. Confidentiality is an absolute obligation that must always be observed.

    D. Trying to negotiate the amount of confidential information that can be shared with other team members is inappropriate behavior.

29. **All the following statements about the interdisciplinary team approach to care are true *except* which one?**

    A. The Medicare Hospice Benefit requires the use of a core team consisting of a physician, a registered nurse, a social worker, and a pastoral or other counselor.

    B. The Medicare Hospice Benefit requires that core members of the team meet at least once every 2 weeks to review each patient's status and care plan.

    C. The team leader bears final responsibility for the team's decisions and has final authority to implement treatment options.

    D. The team is responsible for developing an individualized interdisciplinary plan of care that meets the physical, emotional, social, and spiritual needs of each patient.

30. **All the following statements about interdisciplinary teamwork are true *except* which one?**

    A. The process of decision making is more efficient and takes less time.

B. More effort is needed to communicate effectively and to maintain effective team functioning.

C. Varied professional perspectives may result in comprehensive interventions that meet a patient's physical, social, emotional, and spiritual needs.

D. Shared responsibility may result in a lack of individual responsibility or accountability.

31. **All the following statements about effective teams are true *except* which one?**

A. Effective teams expect team members to assertively represent their discipline's current practice standards.

B. Effective teams recognize and honor the expertise of each team member and carefully evaluate how each discipline can contribute to the patient's and family's well-being.

C. Effective teams expect individual and collective accountability for developing interventions and following through.

D. Effective teams rely on the talents of one experienced team member to provide leadership.

32. **All the following statements about team member roles are true *except* which one?**

A. Role ambiguity, role conflict, and role overload impede individual and team performance.

B. Role ambiguity occurs when roles and expectations are poorly defined and inadequately communicated.

C. Role conflict can be alleviated by listing all the tasks associated with each role and discussing areas of role overlap.

D. Role overload is rarely associated with unrealistic personal expectations regarding job performance or crises in the personal lives of team members.

33. **Which of the following statements about conflict resolution is correct?**

A. Effective facilitators welcome the existence of conflict and view it as an opportunity for positive change.

B. Effective facilitators encourage participants to address all areas of conflict.

C. Effective facilitators concentrate more on long-term goals than on short-term goals.

D. Effective facilitators encourage participants to chose several solutions and implement all of them

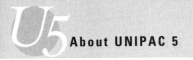

34. **Characteristics of effective team members include which of the following?**

    A. Professional competence and excellent communication skills

    B. Patience, flexibility, and tolerance of ambiguity

    C. Ability to set personal limits and to take responsibility for actions

    D. All the above

35. **All the following statements about a physician's role on the interdisciplinary team are correct *except* which one?**

    A. Attending physicians should provide the admitting diagnosis and prognosis, order medications and treatments, make inpatient and home care visits when needed, provide medical management of conditions unrelated to the terminal illness, and designate an emergency on-call physician.

    B. Hospice medical directors should confirm the terminal diagnosis, determine the medical appropriateness of treatment options and goals, participate in team meetings, consult with attending physicians when necessary, and evaluate patients in home or inpatient settings as needed.

    C. Hospice medical directors should serve as interdisciplinary team leaders, provide leadership during most family conferences, and approve medical, social, spiritual, and psychological interventions.

    D. Hospice medical directors must be doctors of medicine or osteopathy with a current license to practice and to prescribe scheduled drugs.

36. **Signs and symptoms of physician stress overload include all the following *except* which one?**

    A. Anger, irritability, frustration, and tiredness out of proportion to the work that is being done

    B. Overconscientiousness, impaired perspective, and preoccupation with patients

    C. Distancing, intellectualization, and loss of sense of humor

    D. Ability to establish a satisfying balance between professional and home responsibilities

37. **Strategies for managing stress include all the following *except* which one?**

    A. Developing professional skills and setting realistic goals

    B. Making independent decisions and relying on informal decision-making protocols

C. Acknowledging life's imperfections and the impossibility of guaranteeing a perfect outcome for every patient and family

D. Exercising, participating in outside activities for their intrinsic enjoyment, and setting limits on involvement with professional and civic organizations

38. All the following statements about communication skills are true *except* which one?

A. When training to improve nonverbal communication skills, audiotapes are more effective than visual aides.

B. Videotaping interactions with simulated patients and receiving feedback from experienced facilitators are effective means for improving communication skills.

C. Beneficial behavior changes are most likely to occur when skills training is coupled with exercises that enhance personal growth and awareness.

D. Careful discipline is required to develop reliable skills in interviewing and in understanding the meaning of the patient's communications.

[T]o ask physicians and patients to get to know themselves and each other better through conversation will encounter resistance. What has been true for the evolution of mankind has been equally true for the progress of medicine: We have spared no effort to make better tools but we have paid little attention to learning how to communicate better with one another.

—JAY KATZ[1]

Almost invariably, the act of communication is an important part of therapy; occasionally it is the only constituent. It usually requires greater thought and planning than a drug prescription, and unfortunately it is commonly administered in sub-therapeutic doses.

—ROBERT BUCKMAN[2]

In general, the most common problems are caused by relatively simple errors—faults in common courtesy, failures in listening or in acknowledging the patient's needs.

—ROBERT BUCKMAN[3]

Communication and Hospice/Palliative Medicine

In healthcare settings, the goal of any physician–patient interaction is establishing and maintaining effective working relationships that promote healing and mutual trust.[4] Although talk has been described as the main ingredient and fundamental instrument of medical care,[5] just talking is not enough. Instead, physicians must learn to communicate in ways that establish therapeutic relationships and support successful interventions. Effective empathetic communication is the foundation of excellent patient care.[6] It promotes therapeutic relationships and successful interventions by increasing the physician's understanding of the patient's illness and the *person* who is experiencing the illness. Conversely, it helps patients to understand their illness and their options for end-of-life care, which a significant percentage of patients fail to understand.[7]

In hospice/palliative care settings, the two most common elements of communication are:[8]

- Transmitting medical information: sharing news (often bad) with patients and families

- Engaging in therapeutic dialogue: exploring the patient's and family's dealings and deepest concerns

Physicians generally include both medical information and therapeutic dialogue in any patient interview; however, the mix often changes during the course of a serious illness. Initially, transmitting information may predominate, but therapeutic dialogue often becomes much more important as the patient's condition deteriorates and death approaches.[2] Throughout the course of a terminal illness, patients and their family members look to physicians not only for knowledge and technical skill, but also for guidance, reassurance, hope, meaning, and compassionate understanding. The ability to communicate effectively and compassionately is essential because it contributes to the following:[9]

- *Creation and maintenance of therapeutic, interpersonal relationships.* For practitioners of hospice/palliative medicine, the ability to communicate compassionately is particularly important because the patient–physician relationship most often involves a person who is frail, frightened, and vulnerable due to the effects of a terminal illness and a healthy person who possesses specialized knowledge about the illness, its symptoms, and effective palliative treatments. The patient's vulnerability, coupled with the intimacy of physician–patient relationships, imposes stringent ethical demands on both parties and requires trust, honest communication, and compassion.[10]

- *Exchange of information during assessments and decision making.* During the assessment process, physicians need information from patients to establish a diagnosis. When making treatment decisions, physicians require information and guidance to develop a treatment plan that respects the patient's wishes. Likewise, patients need information from physicians to understand their diagnosis and prognosis, to anticipate the illness's likely effects on their future plans, and to participate in developing a treatment plan that reflects their personal values and wishes.

In addition to scientific competence, physicians must demonstrate competence in listening to a patient's life stories and understanding and honoring their meanings.[11] Without effective communication, physicians may inadvertently exacerbate a patient's suffering by focusing only on the disease and ignoring the patient's emotional, spiritual, and social concerns.

Reducing suffering and improving the patient's quality of life (QOL) are the primary goals of hospice/palliative care. Nevertheless, communication devoted to emotional distress, pain, fatigue, and the illness's effects on the patient's daily activities appears to be quite limited during physician visits. Even when patients report serious health-related QOL problems, emotional functioning and fatigue are not addressed up to 54% of the time.[12]

Discussions about end-of-life issues are difficult for anyone to initiate, including physicians.[8,13] Although an average physician conducts approximately 120,000 to 160,000 patient interviews over the course of a career,[14] most physicians receive little or no training in communicating with patients, families, or other healthcare professionals. A survey of 700 physicians attending a symposium on communication at an annual meeting of the American Society of Clinical Oncology indicated that only 6% had received any formal training in breaking bad news and 74% had no strategy in mind when doing so.[15] In the past, physicians were taught to withhold bad news about diagnosis and prognosis in the mistaken belief that such knowledge was inherently harmful. More recently, the results of numerous studies indicate that most patients not only want such information, but also believe it benefits them, even when the news is bad.[16] Initiating discussions of difficult issues earlier in the course of an illness allows patients to make more informed choices. Routinely addressing them throughout the illness can improve palliation of symptoms and provide patients with opportunities to complete the developmental tasks of dying.[13,17]

Physicians may fear harming patients with frank discussions of distressing information, but dealing with painful realities as openly as possible is usually the best approach.[18] Nevertheless, the manner in which bad news is communicated is critical. Physicians should remember that patients vary in their desire for information. Some want all available information about their diagnosis and prognosis, others want the overall picture but not the details, and a few prefer no information. Even highly skilled physicians may have difficulty determining how much information a patient wants to know. A patient's reluctance to discuss troubling issues may result from:

- The need to deny the existence of life-threatening conditions
- The desire to protect themselves, their family members, and their physicians from distressing emotions associated with discussions of poor prognosis
- Subtle, nonverbal cues from the physician indicating such discussions are unwelcome

See Table 1 for general communication guidelines.

Communication and Patient Satisfaction

Poor communication may be the most common contributing factor in requests for bioethics consults and malpractice suits.[3,6,23,24] In a study of malpractice claims, investigators found little correlation between the frequency of claims and the quality of care

Table 1: General Communication Guidelines

- Honest, compassionate, ongoing communication is a central component of hospice/palliative medicine. Communication increases the patient's and family's sense of control and self-worth and establishes healing bonds among patients, families, physicians, and other healthcare professionals.

- The sense of being heard may be the most effective healing agent for dying patients and their family members.[19] Poor communication contributes to suffering because it exacerbates the patient's and the family's sense of isolation, helplessness, and anxiety.

- Although specific techniques can improve communication, the essence of true communication is the ability to enter into therapeutic relationships based on mutual regard, respect, warmth, genuineness, and unconditional acceptance. Such relationships are characterized by empathetic listening, attentiveness, presence, dialogue, and acknowledgment.[20]

- Because stress, pain, and anxiety interfere with a patient's and family's ability to hear and retain information, it is important to alleviate distressing symptoms as soon as possible, establish therapeutic relationships, and repeat information as often as necessary.

- Involving an interdisciplinary healthcare team helps patients and families to voice their suffering through story, art, music, poetry, biography, and ritual.[21]

- Effective palliative medicine depends on honest communication from patients about their symptoms, preferences, and concerns and honest communication from physicians about the disease, the prognosis, and the likely benefits and burdens of treatments.[22]

provided by individual physicians.[25] Instead, they discovered that physicians most likely to be sued were those whose patients:[26,27]

- Felt as if they had been rushed
- Believed they had received little information
- Felt as if their complaints were ignored

In general, patients express two very basic needs:[9]

- The need to know and understand
- The need to feel known and understood

Patient satisfaction may depend more on the perception of adequate sharing of information and emotional support, than on the amount of time a physician spends with a patient. Just the act of sitting down increases patient satisfaction. Studies of cancer patients indicate that patient satisfaction improves when physicians address their concerns and provide information with warmth, interest, and empathy.

Therapeutic communication is important even with a comatose patient. Caregivers should continue to honor the patient's personhood and the possibility that some information may be absorbed by voicing a greeting when entering the room and explaining intended actions, e.g., moving or bathing the patient, straightening sheets, giving medication, or leaving the room.

Communication, Diagnosis, and Treatment

Studies have repeatedly shown that careful histories provide 70% to 80% of the information needed to make most diagnoses. The physical examination contributes an additional 10%. Laboratory or radiographic findings provide only 10% to 15% of needed information.[25,28,29] When taking a history, effective communication is essential for eliciting adequate information about the patient's physical, psychological, social, and spiritual concerns.

Among interpersonal relationships, the doctor–patient relation is one of the most complex ones. It involves interaction between individuals in non-equal positions, is often non-voluntary, concerns issues of vital importance, is therefore emotionally laden and requires close cooperation.

—CHAITCHIK ET AL.[30]

Common Barriers to Effective Communication

See Table 2 for a list of common barriers.

Table 2: Common Barriers to Effective Communication[2,3,8,31]

Cultural Barriers

■ Lack of experience with death

■ Unrealistic expectations of the healthcare system

■ Changes in societal values

■ Changing role of religion

■ Cultural beliefs regarding disclosure of information

Psychological Barriers

■ Patient's fears of:
  Dying
  Physical symptoms
  Psychological effects
  Treatments
  Financial matters
  Changes in roles

■ Physician's fears of:
  Sympathetic pain
  Expressing emotion
  Eliciting an emotional response
  Doing harm
  Illness or death
  Lack of knowledge
  Blame
  Medical hierarchy

■ Family's fears of:
  Physical care and emotional distress
  Financial repercussions
  Role changes

Listening Barriers

■ Judging and evaluating

■ Assumptions

■ Certainty

■ Limited attention span

Organizational Barriers

■ Healthcare environment and reimbursement issues

■ Lack of motivation and standards of performance

■ Lack of organizational support

Language Barriers

■ Medical language

■ Limited language skills

■ Vocabulary

Cultural Barriers

Unless otherwise noted, much of the information in this section is based on Buckman's work.[2,3,8] Because cultural beliefs, values, and expectations regarding healthcare affect communication among physicians, patients, and family members,[32] physicians must be sensitive to cultural barriers such as the following:

- *Experience with death.* In the United States, the 100-year trend toward deaths occurring in institutions rather than homes means that fewer people have witnessed death. When distressing symptoms are adequately controlled, witnessing the death of another person can be reassuring rather than worrisome, as evidenced by decreased anxiety about dying among hospice patients who observed the peaceful death of another hospice patient.[33]

- *Expectations of the healthcare system and quality of life.* In industrialized countries, highly publicized reports of medical breakthroughs and apparently miraculous cures contribute to the public's unrealistic expectations regarding health and illness. Despite a terminal diagnosis, patients may mistakenly expect to return to good health.

- *Values.* Cultural values regarding productivity, youth, physical attractiveness, and material wealth cannot help but affect a patient's sense of self-worth during the dying process. Society's deepest values also inform public policy regarding the availability and quality of care for terminally ill patients.

- *Changing role of religion.* In the United States, increased secularization and religious pluralism contribute to uncertainty among physicians when discussing death with patients. Physicians can no longer assume that patients share similar beliefs about death and immortality, even when belonging to the same religious tradition (see UNIPAC Two).

- *Disclosure of information.* Important cultural differences regarding information diagnosis and prognosis complicate communication. Research indicates major regional differences in physicians' attitudes and beliefs regarding communication at the end of life.[34] Although current trends in the United States favor more disclosure, internationally, the norm is less disclosure.[35] In northern Europe, full disclosure is common, but fewer eastern European patients indicate that they want information about a bad diagnosis.[36] Palliative care specialists in Europe, Canada, and South America agreed that patients with cancer should be informed of their diagnosis and prognosis, that "do not resuscitate" orders should be written, and that they themselves would prefer information if they had terminal cancer.[34] Although 93% of the Canadian physicians stated that at least 60% of their patients would want to know about a terminal diagnosis, only 26% of European and 18% of South American physicians agreed. Similar results were reported when physicians were asked about the percentage of families wanting a patient to be informed about a terminal prognosis.

Even in the United States, cultural beliefs regarding disclosure vary widely. In a study of 800 senior citizens in the United States, 90% of those of European and African American descent claimed that they would want to know about a terminal diagnosis. Only 65% of Mexican Americans wanted to know, and less than 50% of Korean Americans and Native Americans wanted to know.[35]

Disclosure is particularly problematic when cultural beliefs include the magical notion that discussing an event increases the likelihood of its occurrence. Regardless of culture, physicians must respond with empathy and honor a patient's often competing needs to know and deny. At St. Christopher's Hospice, an acclaimed hospice program in England, physicians rarely confront patients with news of a terminal prognosis. Instead, they provide opportunities for patients to ask questions about diagnosis and prognosis, provide some information, then wait for the patient's response before continuing.

Psychological Barriers

Patient's Fear

- *Fear of dying.* Patients are likely to fear the process of dying more than death itself. Fears often focus on uncontrolled symptoms, increased dependency, the sense of becoming a burden to family members and friends, inability to cope, dementia, abandonment, side effects of treatments, existential concerns, and financial losses. In many cases, effective symptom control, adequate information, and ongoing emotional support help to alleviate fears about dying. A patient's need for denial should also be honored.

Physician's Fears

- *Fear of being changed.* When physicians develop therapeutic relationships with patients, they rarely emerge unchanged. Attempting to truly understand a patient's point of view without making evaluative judgments may challenge the physician's own long-held beliefs, which can be frightening. However, physicians with the courage to risk being changed by a patient's insights are likely to experience personal and professional growth.[37]

- *Fear of expressing emotion.* Physicians may underestimate the amount of emotional distress that they are likely to experience while in the presence of someone who is suffering. When faced with a patient's fatal diagnosis, physicians may feel helpless, useless, and out of control. Because they are trained to conceal their feelings of irritation, panic, sorrow, and uncertainty, they may believe that good physicians never experience or express any emotion other than calm certitude. This mistaken notion is particularly unhelpful when providing end-of-life care. Patients rarely criticize physicians whose eyes tear up with emotion when sharing bad news.

Acknowledging sympathetic pain among colleagues helps physicians to cope with feelings of personal inadequacy and guilt generated by the mistaken notion that competent physicians are immune from a patient's suffering. Unless acknowledged, cumulative grief from personal and professional losses may result in emotional distancing from patients.

- *Fear of eliciting an emotional reaction.* When hearing information about a terminal condition, patients and family members may experience shock, anger, or disbelief. They are likely to cry. Physicians, especially those with no training in hospice/ palliative medicine, may fear these normal reactions. Anticipating emotional reactions can help physicians to guide patients and families through the process of dealing with difficult news.

- *Fear of doing harm.* Physicians untrained in communication are likely to fear doing harm to patients by exploring distressing events. However, compassionate communication strengthens therapeutic relationships and encourages honesty.

- *Fear of illness or death.* One study indicated that medical students may fear death more than other students and that practicing physicians fear death even more than medical students do.[38] If true, physicians are likely to avoid situations that force them to confront their own vulnerability, such as interacting with dying patients.

- *Fear of ignorance and lack of knowledge.* An inability to say "I don't know" weakens therapeutic relationships because patients sense the physician's lack of candor and begin to suspect that honesty is not valued.[39] When faced with a diagnosis with which they have little experience, physicians can acknowledge their lack of experience and their plans for learning more. Physicians need to communicate the message, "I don't know, but I will not abandon you, and we will work on this together."

- *Fear of blame.* A physician's fears about blame often focus on:

    Blame by patients when a diagnosis is bad (shoot the messenger)

    Blame by family members (when illness or death occurs, someone must be at fault)

    Blame by colleagues when a patient dies (medical schools inadvertently reinforce the notion that death is a therapeutic failure when they focus solely on curative therapies)

Family's Fears

- *Fear of physical care and emotional distress.* Family members often fear that they will be unable to provide necessary physical care for the patient. They may also

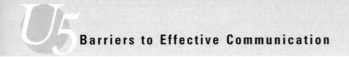

doubt their ability to tolerate the emotional distress that might accompany the dying process.

- *Fear of financial repercussions.* Financial concerns are common. Thirty-one percent of families in the United States lose all or most of their savings during the course of a patient's terminal illness.[40]

- *Fear of role changes.* When one family member becomes terminally ill, the roles of other family members must change to adapt to changed circumstances. Assuming new roles is challenging and often frightening, particularly when the illness necessitates unwelcome changes.

Listening Barriers

White, Kunz, and Hogan described the following listening habits, which act as barriers to effective communication.[41]

Judging and Evaluating

When physicians focus on evaluating and judging instead of listening to what a patient is trying to say, they are likely to miss important information. In difficult and emotional situations, the tendency to evaluate and judge others often increases, which further impedes effective communication at a time when good listening skills are most needed.[37] Instead, physicians must listen carefully for the messages that lie beneath the patient's words.

Assumptions

When physicians make assumptions about a patient's feelings or jump to conclusions about what the patient is going to say next, they lose opportunities to hear important information.

Certainty

Certainty can interfere with the ability to hear new information. For example:

- When convinced that a patient's descriptions of pain are based on drug-seeking behavior, physicians may fail to carefully assess for pain or prescribe effective dosages of medication. (See *UNIPAC Three: Assessment and Treatment of Physical Pain.*)

- When physicians are certain that opioids inevitably depress respirations, they may be unable to hear that individually titrated doses of opioids are the agents of choice for relieving dyspnea in terminally ill patients. (See *UNIPAC Four: Management of Selected Nonpain Symptoms in the Terminally Ill.*)

▪ When physicians are convinced that only certain religious beliefs are correct, they may be unable to effectively address a patient's spiritual concerns. (See *UNIPAC Two: Alleviating Psychological and Spiritual Pain in the Terminally Ill.*)

Limited Attention Span

Effective listening requires the ability to concentrate. A patient's attention span may be limited due to the effects of a terminal illness. A physician's attention span may be limited by concerns about scheduling, which can result in premature closing of interviews or *tuning out* when patients talk about family or social issues.

Organizational Barriers

Healthcare Environment and Reimbursement Factors

The current healthcare environment and reimbursement structure discourage adequate physician–patient communication.[31] Effective communication is likely to require more than the usual 15-minute appointment structure when patients are grappling with news of a fatal diagnosis, poor prognosis, uncontrolled pain, or painful psychological and spiritual issues. In today's cost-conscious healthcare environment, physicians may feel too rushed to (1) take time to establish an ongoing relationship with patients and families, (2) identify psychological, social, and spiritual problems, (3) ensure that patients and family members understand the information being conveyed, and (4) include patients and family members in treatment decisions.

Lack of Motivation and Standards of Performance

Physicians already sensitive to the importance of effective communication are more likely to communicate well and to attend workshops to improve their skills than clinicians most in need of improvement.[31] Linking attendance at workshops and communication performance with an organization's risk management strategy is likely to result in better patient care. Research-based teaching strategies and minimum standards of performance are needed.

Lack of Organizational Support

Encouraging attendance at communication workshops[31] and participation on interdisciplinary teams indicates an organization's support of adequate patient care.

Language Barriers

Medical Language

Physicians speak at least two languages—everyday language and medical language. When physicians try to improve communication by using everyday language, patients and nurses may fail to perceive any change.[9,42] Effective communication depends on the physician's ability to let go of hard-earned medical vocabulary and use words that patients can understand. For example, saying "shot" may be more effective than "injection." "Drip" may be better than "infusion." And "rapid heartbeat" may be more effective than "tachycardia" or "flutter."

Limited Language Skills

In the United States, 14 million patients have limited English language skills. When caring for such patients, healthcare professionals may rely on the patient's family, friends, and neighbors for interpretation.[43] Using nonprofessional interpreters can result in distortions of information and may also:[43,44]

- Undermine patient confidentiality
- Embarrass and inhibit patients
- Expose children to sensitive information
- Subvert family dynamics
- Provide less than complete information
- Result in incomplete histories, ineffective treatments, and inadequate follow-up
- Fail to reveal psychosocial and spiritual concerns

Physicians can improve communication by:[43]

- Using trained interpreters who are truly bilingual
- Providing training on the ethical implications of translating so that interpreters will refrain from changing meanings or ignoring information that they believe will distress the patient or physician
- Providing training on common medical terms, procedures, and prescriptions
- Using bilingual patient educational materials with common expressions, words, and questions
- Learning some basic words and phrases in the patient's language
- Using telephone interpreters; some long-distance carriers provide 24-hour interpretation in all major languages

Vocabulary

Words such as *palliative care, feeding, depression, pain,* and *suffering* are frequently used during end-of-life care, but they are likely to have very different meaning for patients, family members, nurses, physicians, social workers, and chaplains.[45] To improve communication, physicians should choose their vocabulary carefully and explain the terms that they use.

- *Eating or Feeding.* In most people's minds, *eating* refers to the physical act of chewing and swallowing food. *Feeding* refers to spooning food into someone else's mouth. When discussing artificial nutrition, it is better to explain the treatment in nontechnical language and to avoid statements such as "We will continue feeding the patient." The emotional connotations associated with *feeding* interfere with appropriate withdrawal of artificial nutrition or hydration when it no longer serves its therapeutic goal. (See *UNIPAC Six: Ethical and Legal Decision Making When Caring for the Terminally Ill.*)

- *Depression.* Physicians should distinguish the psychiatric condition of depression from everyday feelings of sadness and grief associated with losses related to terminal illness. Patients may exhibit depressive symptoms such as crying, sadness, and sleep difficulties without meeting the DSM IV criteria for depression. (See *UNIPAC Two: Alleviating Psychological and Spiritual Pain in the Terminally Ill.*)

- *Nothing can be done.* This phrase is never helpful. When curative measures are no longer appropriate, intensive symptom control and ongoing, supportive presence are always possible and appropriate. (See *UNIPAC One: The Hospice/Palliative Medicine Approach to End-of-Life Care.*)

- *Hospice care.* Patients, family members, and healthcare professionals may mistakenly associate the word *hospice* with loss of hope, lack of medical care, and uncontrolled pain. Instead, hospice/palliative care focuses on expert symptom control, caring support by a team of compassionate, skilled healthcare professionals, strategies to regain and maintain hope, and joyful living until death occurs. (See *UNIPAC One: The Hospice/Palliative Medicine Approach to End-of-Life Care.*)

Other Barriers

- **Collusion:** The thought of discussing death-related issues can be so anxiety provoking that clinicians, patients, and family members may collude to avoid mentioning death or dying, even when the patient is suffering and the prognosis is poor.[13]

- **Differing agendas:** Patients may want information about their prognosis and the disease's likely impact on their daily lives. Physicians may want to focus on diagnosis and treatment plans.

- **Difficult personalities:** A terminal illness rarely transforms an angry, critical, demanding patient into a gentle effective communicator. Physicians who believe that their technical competence excuses abrupt, uncommunicative behavior are unlikely to become compassionate healers when their patients develop a terminal illness.

- **Structural barriers:** In hospitals, the lack of privacy discourages meaningful communication. Televisions and constant interruptions make sustained conversation difficult. In outpatient settings, cold rooms, rigid schedules, and drafty examination gowns inhibit discussion of troubling issues.

- **Emotional barriers:** Developing therapeutic relationships requires time, emotional energy, and vulnerability. Vulnerability is frightening for most people, especially for physicians, whose training encourages them to demonstrate a sense of authority despite the real uncertainties associated with most medical treatments.

- **Professional barriers:** Historically, physicians have been trained to view the physician–patient relationship as one-dimensional: The physician is the physically healthy, emotionally aloof, adult professional with important knowledge to impart; the patient is a physically ill, often emotional person whose primary role is complying with the physician's orders.[1] The inherent imbalance of power in patient–physician relationships due to differences in health status, expertise, and emotional vulnerability requires special attention to treating patients with dignity, respect, and autonomy. When physicians adhere to a model of shared power and responsibility, they help to establish humane relationships that promote the patient's sense of purpose, value, self-worth, and efficacy. For more information on patient–physician relationships, see *UNIPAC One: The Hospice/Palliative Medicine Approach to End-of-Life Care.* For more information on helping to restore a patient's sense of purpose, value, self-worth and efficacy, see *UNIPAC Two: Alleviating Psychological and Spiritual Pain in the Terminally Ill.*

Understand Nonverbal Communication

Use Effective Nonverbal Communication

At least 70% of interpersonal communication is nonverbal; it is conveyed by tone of voice, eye contact, facial expressions, body position, posture, touch, and physical distance.[46] Patients watch physicians for subtle nonverbal clues communicating the true nature of their condition.[47] When a physicians' nonverbal cues contradict their verbal messages, patients are much more likely to believe the nonverbal cues.[48]

When physicians smile continually and speak rapidly when delivering bad news, they convey their own discomfort, discourage questions, and confuse the patient. Nonverbal signals communicating empathy include:

- Sitting down at eye level with the patient or slightly lower
- Sitting as close to the patient as the relationship dictates
- Sitting in a relaxed position
- Leaning toward the patient

Clarify the Patient's Nonverbal Communication

Because nonverbal cues are culturally influenced[32] and can be difficult to interpret, even experts misinterpret nonverbal cues almost 50% of the time.[48] When a patient's nonverbal communication appears to contradict a verbal message, physicians should ask for clarification.[49,50] For example, when patients say they are feeling fine but their eyes are full of tears, the physician should gently mention the discrepancy, then sit quietly and give the patient a chance to talk about what is really going on. For example, "As we talk, I notice that your eyes are full of tears. Can you tell me something about what you are feeling?" Or "As we talk, I notice that you are looking out the window. Does that mean you are uncomfortable with what we're talking about?"

The meanings assigned to nonverbal communication vary by culture. In general, European cultures view some sustained eye contact as interest. Other cultures, such as the Native American, Asian, and African American cultures, are more likely to view continual eye contact as threatening, hostile, or impolite. When in doubt, following the patient's cues maybe be helpful.[32]

When a patient's nonverbal communication (drawing back, scrunching up, or fidgeting) might indicate discomfort with physical proximity, physicians should move farther away; however, sitting too far away often communicates fear or lack of interest.

AAHPM

Encourage Patients to Talk and Listen to What They Say

Encouraging patients to talk and then listening attentively are critical components of an assessment. As one patient said, "I think it's up to the caregiver, whoever it is, to lead the patient, draw it out of the patient with questions like: What are your concerns? What would you like to know?"[51] In their haste, physicians may do neither; they tend to interrupt patients within the first 18 seconds of an interview and rely on one communication technique—closed questions—that elicit only limited types of information.[52]

The communication strategies described in Table 3 encourage patients to share information about their physical, emotional, social, and spiritual concerns. Listening, acknowledging, clarifying, reassuring, and validating are not just techniques for eliciting information; they also serve as powerful therapeutic interventions because they:[53]

- Create a healing context

- Influence the patient's expectations

- Encourage compliance

- Affect the patient's emotional and physical well-being

- Enable patients to describe not only their physical symptoms, but also their thoughts, feelings, concerns, fears, frustrations, and expectations

Table 3: Effective Communication Strategies[41]

Open-ended Questions

- Open-ended questions give patients permission to describe their symptoms more fully and to say more about what they are thinking and feeling. *Examples:* "Tell me about your pain." "What else can you tell me about where the pain is and how it feels?" "Tell me about your breathing." "Can you tell me more about how you are feeling today?" "Can you tell me something about how your family is coping?" "What are some of the things you want to talk about today?"

- Closed questions rarely elicit additional information, but they are appropriate when patients are exhausted or in pain or when specific information is needed quickly.

Minimal Leads and Accurate Verbal Following

- Minimal leads indicate interest and encourage patients to continue talking; for example, "Uh-huh," "Umm," "Hmm," "Ah."

- Minimal nonverbal leads include nodding the head, eye contact, and leaning toward the speaker.

- Accurate verbal following includes phrases like "Oh?" "Then?" "And?"

Repetition

- Repetition involves repeating one or two key words from the patient's last sentence to indicate that the physician is listening. This encourages the patient to keep talking and enhances the sense of being heard. *Example:* Patient: "When I take the pills I feel nervous." Physician: "The pills make you feel nervous."

- Repetition does not mean the physician agrees with the patient; it only means that the physician is listening.

- Although repetition is an important skill, it should be mixed with other techniques.

Paraphrasing and Reflecting

- When physicians paraphrase and reflect, they repeat a patient's statement in their own words to ensure that the patient's message is understood. *Examples:* "Your medication wasn't delivered until 9 PM; then, when you took the pills, they kept you up all night." Or "When the pain returned, you began to feel anxious and worried." Or "When you think about dying, you worry about uncontrollable pain."

Clarifying Responses

- Clarifying responses help physicians to understand the facts and the patient's feelings and attitudes. *Examples:* "Is it possible that you feel . . . ?" "Can you give me an example of what you are talking about?" "You say you are feeling good *most* of the time; what is going on when you are not feeling well?"

- Clarifying responses also help patients to think about what they have just said, examine their choices, and look at their life patterns. *Examples:* "In the past, how have you coped when sad things happened?" "If you do that, how is it likely to affect your family?"

Confrontation and Honest Labeling

- This technique gently explores uncomfortable subjects, such as distortions of reality or differences between words and actions; it is not an angry demand that patients confront their mortality or any other subject. *Example:* "When you talk about your wife, you say that you understand why she doesn't visit you more often, but I see tears in your eyes. Can you tell me more about how you feel when she doesn't visit?"

Integrating and Summarizing

- These techniques help to ensure that the patient's main concerns are understood. They help physicians and patients clarify their thoughts and feelings and encourage them to further explore confusing issues. *Example:* "Let me see if I understand what you have told me. When the pain returned, you thought it meant you were going to die soon, which made you feel frightened and alone and you thought about ending your life. However, if the pain can be controlled and people come to visit you, you'd rather live a little longer because you have some important things you'd like to do before you die."

Respond with Empathy

- Empathetic relationships are the medium of healing.[53] Empathy refers to the ability to:[2]

  Put aside personal agendas and view the situation from the patient's point of view

  Respond in ways that communicate the physician's awareness and acceptance of the patient's emotions

  Listen to a patient's words, but hear the unspoken messages lying underneath

- When physicians respond with empathy, they create an atmosphere in which patients and family members feel free to voice their deepest concerns without fear of rejection, isolation, or abandonment.

- Empathetic presence helps patients and families to relax into the present moment, which is almost always less frightening than concerns about the past or fears about the future.

- Two of the greatest challenges of empathetic presence are remaining present when the patient's suffering evokes the physician's own fears and insecurities *and* resisting the almost irresistible need to "do something" when listening is the more appropriate action.[54] The greatest test of empathetic presence is being, not doing. ***Don't just do something, sit there!***

- Empathetic response involves following the patient's lead regarding physical contact and remembering that holding a hand or giving a hug can have a strong and lasting positive effect, if done at the right time with the right patient.[55]

- Empathetic physicians are sensitive to the inherently unequal nature of the patient–physician relationship, and they do all that they can to help patients to retain a sense of autonomy and self-worth. (See *UNIPAC One: The Hospice/Palliative Medicine Approach to End-of-Life Care*.)

Example

NOTE: The following anecdote illustrates *lack* of empathy.

Ron is a 62-year-old patient diagnosed with malignant sarcoma 2 years ago and treated with surgery, radiation, and chemotherapy. He has been in remission ever since. Ron also has early cataracts and a history of iodine allergy. One morning Ron begins to cough and goes to the emergency room for chest x-rays, which reveal a right upper lobe mass. His wife, Ann, is a registered nurse at the hospital where her husband is x-rayed. She sees the chest film and fears that her husband is dying. To avoid the implications of the x-ray, Ann focuses all her attention on Ron's cataracts.

The radiologist recommends a CAT scan with contrast, but insists that Ron return home for 24 hours of pretreatment with steroids due to his iodine allergy. Ann refuses the steroids because she is concerned about their effects on her husband's developing cataracts. She contacts her husband's oncologist, who is a friend and professional colleague. The oncologist calls the radiologist, suggests a scan without contrast, and offers to stand by and treat any problems caused by the contrast. The radiologist is furious and yells, "No one is going to tell me how to do my job!"

Ann is very angry when the radiologist once again refuses to perform the scan unless Ron receives pretreatment. The radiologist responds to Ann's distress by defending his professional judgment, credentials, and experience. The oncologist feels trapped in the middle of a very uncomfortable situation that has somehow become worse. Both the radiologist and the oncologist explain to Ann that 24 hours of treatment with steroids will not worsen Ron's cataracts. Ron must suspect something, but none of the involved parties talk with him about the results of the x-ray or inquire about his treatment preferences.

In this case, Ann's colleagues fail to recognize that they are dealing with two frightened people: Ron and Ann. They make the common mistake of continuing to interact with Ann solely as a healthcare professional instead of recognizing that she is a distressed family member in need of support and guidance. The radiologist and oncologist react to their need "to do something" for the husband of a professional colleague, instead of responding to Ann and Ron with empathy and listening for the unspoken messages lying beneath Ann's words.

Use Appropriate Humor

Appropriate humor is a powerful intervention for coping with loss.[56–58] However, sensitivity and intuition are critical when using humor in palliative care settings.[58] Therapeutic humor is distinguished by the following characteristics: it is appropriate and timely, it builds confidence, it brings people together, and it recognizes common dilemmas and paradoxes. It does not ridicule people, destroy confidence, or diminish teamwork.[59]

In his book, *Holyquest: The Search for Wholeness,* Perrino suggests that the nature of true humor lies less in being funny or telling jokes than in kindly contemplation of life's incongruities.[60] According to Perrino, true humor has emotional and spiritual significance because it:

- Relieves tension, punctures pretense, and restores perspective
- Allows the mind to function more effectively and enables people to deal with difficulties more creatively

(AAHPM

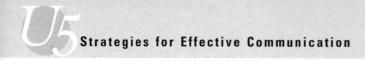
- Enhances a sense of wholeness—when people can laugh at themselves, they are re-reinforcing their identity apart from an event or condition and reflecting their ability to transcend current circumstances

- Enables people to regard life's incongruities with kindly rather than anxious or angry contemplation

- Establishes and preserves a sense of self apart from the vicissitudes of life

Because humor requires perspective, i.e., the ability to step back from a situation and recognize its paradoxical qualities, it is usually possible only when people have confidence in the larger worthwhileness of life. When patients or healthcare providers are suddenly confronted by the deeply tragic aspects of human existence and temporarily engulfed by overwhelming emotions, maintaining a sense of perspective is difficult. Then, attempts at humor are inappropriate. The recovery process is better served by providing calm, ongoing support as patients and professionals search for a renewed and enlarged sense of meaning and purpose. When some sense of perspective is regained, periodic gentle humor and lightheartedness with patients and team members may once again be appropriate.

Dying patients have identified several strategies for maintaining a sense of hope in the face of terminal illness, one of which is a lighthearted approach to situations. Patients also indicate that healthcare professionals may be the only people with whom they can share humor about their situation. "Humor makes me feel that the person knows I'm still alive; if I can laugh, I feel like I still have some power."[61]

Researchers in the field of gelotology, the study of physiological reactions to humorous events, suggest that, in most situations, physical reactions to humor are beneficial. Laughter reduces stress, aids ventilation, accelerates the exchange of residual air, exercises the myocardium, increases arterial and venous circulation, and reduces vascular stasis.[56]

Examples

NOTE: The following anecdotes illustrate the essence of true humor: appreciating life's paradoxes, accepting human frailties, and integrating the often tragic nature of human existence into life without bitterness or sarcasm.

Father and Son. A middle-aged man with a brain tumor was dying in the same manner he had lived his life—cantankerously, irascibly, and continually making mountains out of molehills. When the patient's wife and teenage son returned from the hospital cafeteria, they found him sprawled across his bed, exposing himself, and yelling at the staff. As the patient's wife and son recounted the distressing story to the physician, the son looked up and said, "You know, Dad never was willing to go along with the program." In that moment of insight and acceptance of his father's lifelong frailties, the son helped his mother, the physician, and himself regain a sense of perspective and accept their common dilemma with tolerance, compassion, and humor.

Physician's Family. In the midst of grieving the death of a prominent physician, the bereaved family was able to laugh at the incongruities of life when a friend gently reminded them to schedule the funeral so that it would not conflict with an important football game. The family's appreciation of the friend's concern for their feelings and their ability to step back and recognize the situation's absurdity resulted in tension-reducing laughter, a temporarily renewed sense of perspective, and increased acceptance of the death.

(Conceal) most things from the patient while you are attending to him. Give necessary orders with cheerfulness and serenity, turning his attention away from what is being done to him; sometimes reprove sharply and emphatically, and sometimes comfort with solicitude and attention, revealing nothing of the patient's future or present condition.

—OATH OF HIPPOCRATES (FIFTH CENTURY BCE)[1]

No news is not good news, it is an invitation to fear.

—FLETCHER[62]

Bad news pertains to "situations where there is either a feeling of no hope, a threat to a person's mental or physical well being, a risk of upsetting an established lifestyle, or where a message is given which conveys to an individual fewer choices in his or her life."

—BOR ET AL[63]

An expert in breaking bad news is not someone who gets it right every time—he or she is merely someone who gets it wrong less often, and who is less flustered when things do not go smoothly.

—BUCKMAN[3]

Communicating bad news is generally regarded as one of the most difficult tasks of medicine. However, studies indicate that patients usually prefer to have information about their diagnosis and prognosis, even when the news is worse than expected.[64] Physicians may fear harming patients by communicating the truth, but most patients report positive results of being told bad news, for example, having a label for their condition, which explains their symptoms and reduces their sense of uncertainty. When bad news about diagnosis and prognosis is withheld, patients are more likely to experience the following:[65]

- Distress when the diagnosis is learned by accident
- Confusion when told the diagnosis by someone other than the physician in charge
- A sense of being patronized when physicians withhold important information

- Feelings of loneliness and isolation when they sense that something is very wrong but cannot talk about it

- Disruption when family members know the diagnosis and prognosis but the patient does not

- A loss of trust in professional and family caregivers

Because judgments about the "badness" of news are subjective, physicians should avoid making assumptions about how bad news will affect a patient. For example, a patient may be relieved to hear a diagnosis of cancer instead of amyotrophic lateral sclerosis. Nevertheless, bad news is emotionally distressing for recipients. Therefore, the manner in which it is communicated is vital. Empathy may be the distinguishing characteristic between clinicians perceived as providing comfort when delivering bad news and those whose manner causes further distress. Often the only palatable aspect of hearing bad news is the physician's deep concern about the news and empathy with the patient's plight: "This must be terrible for you; we will work on it together." Table 4 describes patients' preferences when physicians share distressing news.

Hospice/palliative physicians rarely have to communicate bad news about a terminal diagnosis. More often, they communicate bad news about the meaning of changes in the patient's condition; for example, the patient has entered the *terminal* phase of what may have been a chronic illness. In many cases, patients with terminal diseases, such as breast cancer, prostate cancer, congestive heart failure, HIV/AIDS, or emphysema, have coped fairly well for several years. Now, possibly for the first time, they are faced with the full implications of their condition.[66,67]

Table 4: Patients' Preferences When Physicians Communicate Bad News[62]

- Direct, empathetic communication
- Information about diagnosis, which provides a label for their condition
- Information about prognosis and how the illness is likely to affect their quality of life
- Inclusion of a family member or trusted friend in the discussion
- Encouragement to ask questions
- Information that is neither overly optimistic nor overly pessimistic
- Practical information about what to do and how to obtain additional information

---

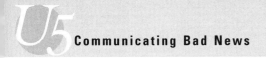

General Guidelines for Communicating Bad News

Table 5 includes general guidelines for communicating bad news.

Table 5: General Guidelines for Communicating Bad News[36]

- Disclosing information should not be a one-time event; instead, communication should be an ongoing process whose pace is determined by the patient's personality, coping mechanisms, and desire to know more.

- Studies indicate that physicians, nurses, and other team members consistently underestimate the amount of information that patients want and misinterpret the kinds of information that they desire. Physicians often want to talk about diagnosis and treatment, but patients more often want information about the disease's likely impact on themselves and on their family members, how their prognosis is likely to affect their future plans, psychological issues related to their diagnosis and prognosis, and practical information about available resources to cope with daily living.

- Most patients with a terminal illness know that they are dying; avoiding discussions of prognosis is likely to increase their sense of loneliness and abandonment and deny them opportunities for meaningful communication about death-related issues. Some patients may prefer ambiguous information that allows them to continue hoping for a cure, but, in most cases, lack of information only increases stress and anxiety, particularly when patients suspect the true diagnosis.

Effective Strategies for Communicating Bad News

Several helpful protocols for communicating bad news are available.[2,8,68] In any case, compassion and caring human presence are the essential components of communicating such news.

Six-Step Protocol for Communicating Bad News[2]

1. Arrange the physical context and the emotional atmosphere.

2. Find out how much the patient knows.

3. Find out how much the patient wants to know.

4. Share information (align and educate).

5. Respond to the patient's feelings.

6. Make a plan and follow through.

Plan Carefully and Arrange the Physical Context

Planning takes a few minutes but it saves time and distress in the long run, particularly when bad news must be shared and the patient's reactions are likely to be emotional.

Prepare for the Interview

- Prior to the interview, review the medical facts of the case, any major concerns previously voiced by the patient or family, and relevant family dynamics.

Arrange the Interview Structure

- Arrange for an unhurried, uninterrupted time in a private room or the patient's home, where patients and family members can ask questions and express themselves freely.

- Turn pagers to a nonaudible setting and reroute telephone calls if possible.

- Include a family member or friend in the interview for the following reasons:

    The patient feels less alone and has someone to talk with after the physician leaves.

    The friend or family member can help to provide support for the patient and serve as a witness to what was actually said and how the news was delivered.

    The physician has an opportunity to model open and compassionate communication about death and dying and can help to prepare friends and family for the patient's death.

    When no family member or friend is available, including a nurse or other team member in the interview is helpful for many of the same reasons.

Arrange the Physical Environment

- Arrange the physical environment so that physical barriers such as bedside tables and trays do not interfere with verbal and nonverbal communication. Televisions and radios should be turned off.

- Arrange seating so that it encourages communication: the physician should sit close enough to the patient to attend to the patient's emotional responses and provide therapeutic touch when needed and appropriate. A distance of 2 to 3 feet is usually comfortable for personal discussions, but follow the patient's cues; some patients may need more or less personal space. If possible, place the physician's chair at right angles to the patient's instead of behind a desk or across the room.[69]

- Make sure facial tissues are within everyone's reach.

Arrange the Emotional Atmosphere

Establish a Caring Relationship

Make Introductions

- Acknowledge the presence of all parties, determine their relationships, and introduce everyone in the room, including other healthcare professionals.

- Shaking hands is a matter of cultural and personal preference. If cultural norms support hand shaking, shake the patient's hand first if possible, even when other family members are present.

Sit Down

- *This is the most important rule and should always be followed, even when chairs must be brought from another room.*

Assess the Patient's Knowledge and Emotional Response

- Before communicating bad news, find out what information has already been shared with the patient, the patient's impression of the seriousness of the illness, how the illness is currently affecting the patient's daily life, and the patient's understanding of the likely prognosis. Answers to these questions can help physicians to decide what information to share first and how to share it. After asking a question, stop and give the patient plenty of time to answer. Buckman suggests the following questions:[2]

What has the doctor told you about your illness?

What did Dr. X tell you when you were referred for hospice/palliative care?

What does that mean to you?

How serious does your illness seem to be?

Did you think something serious was going on when . . . ?

▪ Patients may say that other physicians have told them nothing about their illness, but anxiety and denial often interfere with a patient's ability to hear and retain information. When physicians are aware that patients have been told information and are now denying it, they should communicate as if the patient had no previous knowledge. Confronting patients or expressing amazement or concern about their lack of knowledge or the communication habits of other physicians is not helpful.

▪ Identify the emotions that the patient and family are experiencing, and respond in ways that convey respect for these feelings. Even patients (especially healthcare professionals) who respond in a highly intellectual manner are likely to be experiencing feelings of deep anxiety and fear. Buckman suggests questions such as:[2]

What has worried you the most about this situation? What else has worried you?

How worried have you been about yourself?

It must be distressing for you that the therapy has not resulted in a longer remission.

Assess How Much the Patient Wants to Know

▪ Discovering how much patients want to know is an important part of the communication process. Although patients have a right to the full disclosure of truthful information and most desire it, some do not. Gently ask patients how much they want to know, and remind them that they can end the interview whenever they need to. A follow-up interview can be rescheduled after they have had a chance to assimilate the news. Be sensitive to the patient's needs and consider questions such as those recommended by Buckman and others:[2]

I want to talk with you about your illness, but I'm not sure what you want to know. Sometimes people want to know all the details about their condition and sometimes they just want to know the big picture. What do you want?

AAHPM

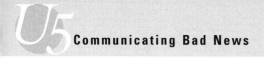
What is the most important information for you to have now?

Do you want to hear the basic facts now and then talk more at a later time?

Will you let me know when you want to stop talking so that we can resume our discussion after you've had a chance to think about it?

Share Information

Physicians often underestimate a patient's desire for knowledge and may spend little more than 1 minute of a 20-minute interview sharing information.[70] Effective communication takes time. It requires the following: tailoring information to the patient's needs, determining the patient's understanding of what has been said, and clarifying misunderstandings.

Use Plain Language

- Promise to answers questions openly and honestly.

- Choose vocabulary carefully, and use simple, everyday language (no medical jargon, euphemisms, or technical, diagnostic terminology).

- Use the patient's factual understanding and style of communication to guide information sharing. When medical terminology is required or requested by patients or families, first explain the medical terms in everyday language.

- Encourage patients and family members to take notes. Some physicians suggest that patients record conversations so that they can refer to the tape later; however, medical or legal concerns may present challenges to recording conversations.

Adapt to the Patient's Style

- Use the same general vocabulary as the patient. Use caution when communicating with patients who use medical language; their understanding of the terminology may be faulty. Remain cautious when communicating with patients who are healthcare professionals; their emotional responses are like those of any other patients, and they are likely to experience similar difficulties hearing and retaining distressing information.

Fire Warning Shots When Needed

- When large gaps exist between the patient's knowledge and medical reality, verbal messages should indicate that the situation is more serious than the patient realizes. For example, "I'm afraid the situation is more serious than we thought."

Share Information in Small Steps

▪ Provide information gradually, allow patients to determine the pace at which they are told information, and listen carefully for their need for denial.

▪ Gradually bring the patient's understanding closer to medical reality.

▪ Remember that stress interferes with the ability to hear and retain information. Physicians may need to repeat information several times during the course of the interview and during the next several days, weeks, or months.

▪ Let the patient's reactions dictate how much they are told.

Stop Frequently

When sharing information, stop frequently to assess for:

▪ **The patient's understanding of what has been said and misinformation that needs to be corrected.** Example: "This must be very confusing. Am I making sense? Can you tell me what you understand so far, so I'll know what to talk about next?"

▪ **The patient's emotional response to what has been said.** Notice body language and ask patients about their responses to the news. Try not to make assumptions about how the news is affecting them. Example: "Can you tell me something about how this information is affecting you?"

▪ **Unspoken concerns that have not yet been addressed.** Ask patients and family members if they have questions that have not yet been answered; then pause long enough to let them formulate questions. Example: "This must be very difficult for you. What are some of the questions or concerns we haven't addressed yet?"

▪ **The patient's ability to continue listening.** After hearing the word *cancer*, patients may not hear another word. When patients are no longer listening, stop and schedule another interview. Continued attempts to communicate will be unproductive. Example: "This must be very confusing and overwhelming. Do you want to spend some time thinking about what we've discussed so far, then get back together later?"

Provide Information That Patient Wants to Know

▪ Physicians and patients often have different goals when sharing information. Physicians tend to emphasize medical information about the disease, e.g., its stages and possible treatments. Patients often want this information, but they also want information about prognosis and how the symptoms will affect their everyday lives. For example, they want to know how long they will live and how much pain they will have.[30] Try to elicit as many of the patient's concerns as possible.

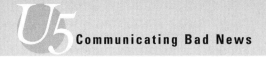

Provide Information about Prognosis

When patients seek information about prognosis, physicians may feel torn by at least three competing needs:

- They want to communicate honestly so that patients can make decisions about how to spend their remaining time.

- They want to avoid harming patients and fear that truthful communication about limited prognosis may destroy hope.

- They want to avoid discussions about poor prognoses due to their own discomfort with the topic.

Patients and family members have legitimate needs for information about prognosis, including the need to prioritize their plans for the future. Most family members want to be at the patient's side when death occurs and will temporarily abandon all other plans when death appears to be imminent. When patients die unexpectedly and alone, families may feel guilty, but they are usually comforted when healthcare professionals explain that dying patients often appear to choose their time of death. Some patients die just before family members arrive or just after they have left, possibly to protect them from further distress.

When physicians make precise estimates of length of life, the estimates tend to become fixed sentences and, as most physicians know, they often are proved wrong. Nevertheless, patients and families may want and need general information about probable life expectancy.

When patients first ask about the amount of time that they have left, instead of immediately responding with specific time frames, physicians should ask for clarification. Clarification often results in questions that can be answered with more certainty. For example: Patient: "How long have I got?" Physician: "What is your main concern?" Patient: "I want to go fishing again; should I go now?" or "I want to say good-bye to my son; should I call him now?" or "Will I be around when my grandchild is born? Until Christmas? Until I graduate from high school?"[71]

While acknowledging that no one can accurately predict the future, physicians can encourage patients to revise unrealistic goals, go on trips while they are feeling well enough to do so, visit with family, and say and do all the things that they want to accomplish before dying. Such responses convey important information, maintain hope, and encourage patients to complete the developmental tasks of dying.[72] (See *UNIPAC Two: Alleviating Psychological and Spiritual Pain in the Terminally Ill.*)

When patients want more precise information, physicians should provide estimates while remaining aligned with the patient psychologically by acknowledging that:

- All estimates are uncertain.

- People may live longer or shorter than average estimates.

- This particular patient may live longer or shorter than average estimates. For example: Patient: "How long have I got?" Doctor: "No one can predict life expectancy exactly. There is always a lot of uncertainty. Most people with your condition live longer or shorter than a predicted average. We can't say for sure how your disease will progress. But, based on the medical indications and your situation, you are likely to live for a few more weeks and maybe as much as a couple of months."

The important points to remember are:

- Avoid lying. Give patients and families a general time frame that is as accurate as possible.

- The best prognostic indicator usually is the patient's activity level and ability to perform activities of daily living.[73] See UNIPAC One.

- Encourage patients and families to use their remaining time to complete important tasks. (See *UNIPAC Two: Alleviating Psychological and Spiritual Pain in the Terminally Ill.*)

Respond with Empathy

Elicit and Respond to the Patient's Feelings

- Eliciting, acknowledging, and validating a patient's feelings about diagnosis and prognosis are important aspects of effective communication.[9]

- Patients may respond to bad news with stunned silence, anger, disbelief, acute distress, intellectualization, or guilt.[74] When intense distress occurs, physicians sometimes fear that the patient's emotions will remain uncontrollable. In most cases, the best response is to wait quietly until emotions subside, generally within 5 to 10 minutes.

- When patients begin to cry, try not to distract them by immediately patting them, handing them a tissue, or otherwise interfering. Stay calm, let them experience their emotions, and wait until their body language indicates that they are ready for a tissue or a touch. Patients value physicians who can cope with emotional reactions without embarrassment or fear.

- When patients respond with anger, let them speak without responding defensively or trying to correct misconceptions. Anger is usually the result of displaced fear or feelings of being ignored or devalued. When emotions subside, suggest approaches for the problems that can be fixed. When problems cannot be fixed (e.g., death is inevitable), *provide reassurance that the patient will not be abandoned, the physician will concentrate on alleviating symptoms, and the entire team will continue providing support and caring presence.*

- Examples of empathetic responses recommended by Buckman include these: "It must be hard to accept that the illness has taken a turn for the worse when you've been feeling so well," or "This must be overwhelming for you," or "This must be confusing; there is so much to know and so many choices," or "This must be awful for you."

Use Appropriate Self-disclosure

- When used appropriately, self-disclosure can be an effective communication tool as long as the patient's concerns, not the physician's own emotional needs, remain the primary focus. Effective self-disclosure depends on the depth of the physician–patient relationship. During a first interview, appropriate self-disclosure may be limited to acknowledging having lived in the same town or sharing a similar hobby. As the relationship continues, physicians can respond to cues indicating that the patient wants a deeper, more human encounter, as long as professional boundaries are maintained. The following examples illustrate appropriate self-disclosure:

  Acknowledging the physician's feelings: After several weeks of home visits from her physician, an elderly hospice patient commented on the physician's tie, saying it was much more conservative than usual. She guessed he would be attending a meeting. The physician complimented her astute observation and acknowledged that he was on his way to a business meeting. When the patient noted that the physician's tone of voice indicated that he was not looking forward to the meeting, the physician laughed and agreed. These few comments established a more personal connection between the patient and her physician while maintaining appropriate professional boundaries; i.e., the physician did not go on to complain about the grave differences of opinion he was having with a managed care organization.

  Acknowledging feelings in common: When a terminally ill patient's sister commented on the extreme anger she was experiencing as a result of her brother's illness, the physician responded, "When my brother died, I was angry too. How is the anger affecting you and your relationships with your family?" The physician's response aligned the physician with the sister and acknowledged the validity of her feelings, then redirected the focus of the conversation back to her.

Use Therapeutic Silence

▪ Therapeutic silence is an important part of effective communication. When patients suddenly become quiet, they may be experiencing emotions so strong that they are unable to speak. Physicians should stop, remain quiet for a moment, then inquire about what the patient is thinking and feeling. Until emotional needs are assessed and attended to, patients will be unable to hear further information. Example: "This must be difficult to hear. Can you tell me something about what you are thinking and feeling?"

▪ Therapeutic silence allows patients and family members to:

Think about what has been said

Assimilate information

Identify and experience feelings

Integrate their intellectual knowledge and emotional needs

Formulate and ask questions

Use Touch Appropriately

▪ In many cases, touching patients provides them with a sense of reassurance and emotional support. A hug or holding hands can have positive and lasting effects if done with the right patient at the right time.[75] However, physicians must be sensitive to a patient's nonverbal cues about touch. Some patients welcome a touch or a hug, while others are uncomfortable with any touching.

▪ The following nonverbal body language often indicates that the patient is comfortable with touch and finds it reassuring: leaning toward the physician, continuing to hold the physician's hand when it is offered, and leaning into a hug instead of withdrawing. Nonverbal body language indicating discomfort with touch includes quick withdrawal when the physician touches the patient's hand, stiffened body muscles when the physician attempts to touch or hug the patient, and insisting on extreme physical distance.

▪ Empathetic physicians are particularly sensitive to the inherent inequalities of the patient–physician relationship. They understand that rules about touching are very personal and culturally determined[32] and change depending of the nature of the relationship. When a physician and patient are friends, hugging may be appropriate when they meet in social situations. However, when the same patient visits the physician in a professional capacity, the relationship changes and so do the rules about touching. The relationship is now unequal, and the same types of affectionate touching that were appropriate in social settings may not be appropriate. Restraint and careful evaluation of the patient's nonverbal communication are necessary to determine which types of touching are appropriate and therapeutic.

Provide Reassurance, Support, and Hope

- Avoid meaningless statements, such as "Everything is going to be fine." Appropriate reassurance reflects reality, for example: "We will work together on this." "We will do everything we can to control your pain, nausea, breathlessness, etc. If we run into problems, we will call on other consultants for help." "We will do everything we can to make sure you can stay at home."

- Understand that a patient's focus of hope is likely to change during the course of an illness and often increases with effective palliative care.[61] See *UNIPAC Two: Alleviating Psychological and Spiritual Pain in the Terminally Ill.*

- Before the interview ends, explain to the patient and family the process that they should follow for contacting the physician or person on call when they need more information or want to talk. Provide a business card and share telephone numbers. This is particularly important when the interview closes prematurely or when patients are unwilling to discuss important issues.

Make a Plan for the Future and Follow Through

- Most patients and families want their physicians to help them to make sense of the diagnosis and prognosis and to provide guidance when making decisions. Problem-solving approaches involve patients and families in the planning process and reinforce their sense of control and competence. Buckman describes the following five-step process:[3,8]

  1. Help patients and families to identify specific problems; demonstrate understanding of the patient's list of concerns.

  2. Distinguish fixable problems from unfixable ones (pain can be controlled but death cannot be avoided).

  3. Help patients and families to make a plan, while acknowledging uncertainties about the future.

  4. Help patients and families to identify successful coping strategies.

  5. Help patients and families to identify other resources and sources of support.

Summarize the Interview

- Summarize the interview verbally and in written form, if possible.

- Ask for remaining questions, and suggest that patients and families keep a list of questions for the next interview.

Make a Contract and Follow Through

- Making a contract can be as simple as saying, "I will see you in a week or two." In the home care setting, the contract may be "The home care team will be visiting you frequently. Let them know about any problems that you are experiencing and tell them any other concerns that you may have. Call the hospice/palliative care program if you have questions and I will get back to you as soon as I can." Be sure to follow through with promises to return calls promptly.

Although the individual is the unit of treatment, the family is the unit of understanding.

According to family systems theory, each system or subsystem is always part of a larger system, whether it begins with the cardiovascular system, the whole body system, the whole person system, or the whole family system. Each of these systems, or subsystems, is in constant interaction will all other smaller subsystems that are within it, as well as in constant interaction with the larger suprasystem of the environment that is around it.

—WILLIAMSON AND NOEL[53]

Family Systems Theory

Instead of viewing a person as an individual unit, family systems theory views "the individual as one part of a larger (emotional) system of the family, with the family seen as the whole."[53] Family systems theory suggests that a patient's actions are best understood within the context of the family system, which sets rules about communication and interaction. The basic concepts of family systems theory include:[53]

- The whole is greater than the sum of the parts. For example, a person is more than the sum of various bodily systems.

- Whatever affects the system as a whole affects each part. For example, the effects of morphine affect not only the sensory system, but also the gastrointestinal and cognitive systems and the patient's ability to interact with family and friends.

- A change in any part of a system affects every part of the system *and* the system as a whole. For example, pain relief positively benefits not only the patient, but also the entire family system.

Regardless of a system's size or complexity (whether it is a single individual, a family, or an interdisciplinary team), systems are dynamic. They develop rules, roles, and patterns of behavior to sustain themselves. Because systems tend to view any change as a threat to their continued existence, they fear even beneficial changes and rely on entrenched behavior patterns, even when those behaviors are no longer helpful.

Family systems must constantly adjust to internal stressors (e.g., the birth of a child or a serious illness) and external stressors (e.g., job loss, cultural or religious discrimination, lack of access to health care). When profound stressors occur, such as a terminal illness and death of a family member, the entire family system is thrown out of balance. The stresses associated with adaptation may trigger or exacerbate long-standing family issues related to beliefs, roles, rules, and unresolved earlier losses.

The Family Life Cycle

Like any other system, families experience developmental stages, such as the following:

- New couple
- Family with young child(ren)
- Family with adolescent(s)
- Family with children leaving home
- Aging family dealing with retirement and the death of one parent, then the other

Whether changes are expected and welcomed (birth of child) or unexpected and feared (job loss, divorce, or serious illness), they require major adjustments in the family's roles and functions. When the death of a family member occurs in the midst of a new developmental stage, the combined stress of adjusting to the death and the developmental stage is likely to pose tremendous challenges for the entire family system.

Family Interaction Models

Enmeshed or Disengaged

Minuchin describes family systems as *enmeshed* or *disengaged*.[76] When families are enmeshed, their tightly woven relationships present an almost impenetrable barrier to the outside world. The identities of enmeshed family members are so interconnected with each other and with the family system as a whole that the death of one member creates particularly difficult identity and self-esteem problems for survivors. Enmeshed families may find it difficult to communicate with or accept help from outsiders due to unspoken rules prohibiting the sharing of information with strangers.

Disengaged families represent the other extreme. They are so separate from one another that there is little mutual dependence, little sharing of functions and roles, and limited emotional support. Family bonds may appear nonexistent, and team members may have difficulty distinguishing family members from visitors and friends. However, when serious illness occurs, disengaged families may temporarily regroup and erect barriers between the family and the outside world.

The terms *enmeshed* and *disengaged* do not always imply dysfunction. All families exist somewhere on a continuum of enmeshed and disengaged interaction according to the family's needs. Functional enmeshment is appropriate in certain situations; for example, when an infant is born, the tightly woven interdependent connections between the parents and the child help to ensure the child's survival. When a family member is dying, family members often assume the patient's responsibilities and provide much more physical and emotional support than usual, thus protecting the patient until death occurs.

Closed or Open

Satir describes family systems as *open* or *closed*, depending on the family's communication patterns, rules, and relationships with the outside world.[77] An open family system's permeable boundaries and encouragement of supportive relationships with the outside world generally allow greater access to patients and family members. Closed family systems, like other closed groups, whether they are social, religious, or work related, establish rigid boundaries between their members and outsiders, presenting challenges for hospice/palliative care teams. Table 6 describes the characteristics of open and closed family systems.

Although open family systems often are better able to adapt to changing situations than closed family systems, open families also experience tremendous stress as members adapt to the terminal illness and death of a family member. For physicians, the important point to remember is that a family's beliefs and patterns of behavior influence:

- Its willingness to ask for and accept help
- Its ability to communicate about illness and death
- Its willingness to care for the dying person
- Its response to the death of one of its members

Family Subsystems

Within families, smaller subsystems exist based on age (adults or children), sex (mothers and daughters), areas of interest (reading or fishing), or function (subgroups of grandparents, parents, or siblings). Other family subsystems include the following:[41,77]

- **Pairs:** Each pair has a role name, such as husband–wife, mother–son, husband–son, mother–daughter, etc. Families with rigid beliefs (rules) are likely to experience particular difficulty when confronted with change, e.g., a strict belief that only wives cook leads to adjustment difficulties when the wife becomes too ill to cook.
- **Triangles:** Families with more than two members contain subsystems of triangles. A family of five members includes thirty triangles: father–mother–first son, father–mother–daughter, father–first son–daughter, etc. Due to the number of triangles

Table 6: Characteristics of Open and Closed Family Systems[77]

Open	Closed
Characteristics	

Open

Characteristics

- Views change as normal, inevitable, and desirable.
- Encourages supportive relationships with the outside world.
- Uses direct, clear, and specific communication.
- Uses flexible rules to govern the family's behavior.
- Encourages communication and comments about family rules and beliefs.
- Self-worth is primary; power and performance are secondary.
- Actions represent one's beliefs.

Rules and Beliefs

- Mistakes are normal and OK.
- Feelings are important.
- We can work it out.
- You are a special person.
- It is OK to ask for what you want.
- We can talk about our problems with each other and with the outside world.

Closed

- Change is feared and resisted.
- Restricts contact or transactions with the outside world.
- Uses indirect, unclear, and nonspecific communication.
- Uses covert rules that don't change according to family needs.
- Prohibits comments about family rules and beliefs.
- Self-worth is secondary to power and performance.
- Actions are subject to the whims of the "boss."

- Never make mistakes.
- Don't raise your voice.
- Don't talk about _____'s illness or death.
- Children must be protected from painful experiences, e.g., funerals.
- Asking for what you want is selfish.
- We can't talk about or acknowledge our family secrets.
- Relationships have to be regulated by force or punishment.
- There is one right way, and the person with the most power is the only one who knows it.
- Those in authority know what is best for you.

existing in each family, dysfunctional relating challenges the entire family system; e.g., when parents experience relationship difficulties, one of them may turn to a child or to an outside affair for emotional support instead of seeking professional help or talking with friends.

- **Coalitions:** Coalitions are subsystems that form to serve a special purpose. During a terminal illness, they commonly form around issues such as the location of care; e.g., one coalition may insist that the patient remain at home, while another insists that the patient move to a nursing facility.

Family Responses to Terminal Illness and Death

A family system's response to the profound illness and death of one of its members is affected by the system's beliefs and behavior patterns, including family roles, rules, and level of intimacy.

Family Roles

When one member of a family system becomes profoundly ill or dies, other family members must assume new roles and responsibilities. The amount of disruption experienced by the family system is likely to be affected by the following:[41]

- **Family position held by the individual.** If the individual is the family's only child, the parents will experience tremendous stress as they adjust to a state of childlessness.

- **Number and type of roles held by the individual.** If the individual is the family's only wage earner or the family's main communicator, remaining family members are likely to experience significant stress as they learn to cope with financial issues or to communicate directly with one another instead of through the communicator.

- **Ability of family members to perform tasks essential to family life.** If illness, handicap, or lack of education and skills interferes with the family's ability to fill a vacant role, the system will experience significant stress until family members adjust or find outside help.

- **Degree of scapegoating.** Dysfunctional families often identify one family member as the problem person and blame that person for all the family's problems. By focusing on problems caused by the scapegoat instead of on its own systemic problems, the family tries to avoid change, a much-feared process that could result in the "death" of dysfunctional but familiar behavior patterns.

Family Rules

When one member of a family system becomes profoundly ill, adjustments in family rules usually are required. For example, a family rule against accepting outside help must be adapted if the family is to receive financial help from the Medicare Hospice Benefit. The ill-conceived drug-abuse prevention slogan "just say no" may result in family rules prohibiting drug use that must be adapted if the patient requires medication to relieve pain. A rule prohibiting outsiders in the home must be adapted to allow home care.

Intimacy Patterns

- **Isolation:** When death occurs, family members may become so isolated in their own grief that they are unable to emotionally support themselves or other members of the family. Then the family system requires temporary support from a bereavement team until adequate functioning is restored.

- **Changes in relationship patterns:** The stresses associated with a terminal illness and death may strengthen emotional ties among family members, but the stresses can also cause disintegration of family relationships. Families may temporarily change their pattern of relating during the illness, but are likely to revert to their former patterns after the death occurs.

- **Touch:** Patients vary in their need for touch. Some seriously ill patients suffer from a lack of touching and want the emotional reassurance and healing that caring touch provides. Others do not want to be touched.

Protracted illness and inpatient care often interfere with a couple's privacy needs. Some couples want privacy for long talks, cuddling, prayer, or sexual intimacies. Physicians should encourage them to establish private times, particularly during inpatient stays. Other couples are distressed by intimacy and fear the personal aspects of home care. Such patients may not want family members, including spouses, to touch them or provide personal care. In any case, the patient's wishes should be respected.

Facilitating Family Conferences

Direct physician contact with patients and their families is necessary, particularly when catastrophic illness and/or death challenges a family system.[78,79] Physician participation in family conferences is an essential component of caring. To participate effectively, physicians should understand the basics of family system theory, develop a sense of the family's beliefs and behaviors, and recognize the family's current stage of development.

CAAHPM

Careful planning is essential for effective family conferences. Prior to the conference, the physician should confer with other members of the interdisciplinary team and decide the following:

- Which family members and professional staff will participate in the conference?
- Do individual issues exist that must be addressed one-to-one prior to the conference?
- Will the patient participate in the conference? If not, why not?
- Where and when will the conference take place? Which room can comfortably accommodate participants? What time is most convenient for family members?
- Which professional staff will assume responsibility for various aspects of the conference; e.g., who will invite family members? When the conference begins, who will review the ground rules?

Use Counseling Techniques

When physicians work with patients and families, their primary responsibility is to perform the following tasks with empathy and careful attention to detail:

- Examine the patient (complete a history and physical).
- Help patients and families to understand the suspected diagnosis and prognosis.
- Help patients and families to make sense of what is happening to them.
- Present and explain a suggested medical treatment plan and negotiate with the patient and family until a mutually acceptable plan is established.
- Work with a team to develop an interdisciplinary treatment plan.
- Provide ongoing guidance and emotional support.

Most terminally ill patients and family members are not looking for prolonged or formal psychotherapy from their physicians. Instead, they want information and guidance so that they can make sense of what is happening to them. They also want support as they search for a renewed sense of purpose, meaning, value, and hope. Table 7 lists basic counseling techniques that physicians can use during family conferences to elicit the patient's and family's concerns and to provide appropriate support. Although physicians have immediate medical responsibility to the patient, during family conferences physicians are most effective when they maintain equal loyalty to all members of the family.[53]

On occasion, physicians encounter patients and family members whose deep-seated problems clearly exceed the physician's skills. Appropriate actions include requesting involvement of team members with specialized counseling skills and consulting with team

> ### Table 7: Counseling Techniques for Physicians to Use During Family Conferences
>
> - Use listening techniques and nonverbal behaviors that communicate empathy and interest, encourage patients and family members to talk, indicate that the physician is listening, and enhance the patient's and family's sense of being heard. (See Strategies for Effective Communication on pages 33–39.)
>
> - Demystify and correct misconceptions, such as "the use of morphine causes addiction" or "when artificial nutrition is withheld, terminally ill patients suffer and their lives are shortened." (See UNIPACs Three, Four, and Six.)
>
> - Acknowledge the family's fear, grief, and guilt; e.g., "If only I had fed him more, he wouldn't be so thin." "If only I had taken her to a different doctor, she wouldn't be dying now."
>
> - Exhibit equal loyalty to all members of the family, and refrain from taking sides with one or more family members.[1]
>
> - Help patients and family members to identify their strengths and set realistic short-term goals.
>
> - Use reframing to help patients and families to recognize other perspectives.
>
> - Help patients and families to make sense of what is happening to them by engaging them in an ongoing search for meaning. (See *UNIPAC Two: Alleviating Psychological and Spiritual Pain in the Terminally Ill.*)

members about referrals to outside sources for specialized counseling and/or psychiatric treatment.

Anticipate Problems and Mediate Conflict

Patients and family members may differ in their expectations of hospice/palliative care and the goals of treatment. Effective mediation helps to resolve conflicts because it:[80]

- Involves a third party

- Increases the participants' sense of being heard and clarifies their views and attitudes

- Reduces defensiveness and exaggerated positions and statements

- Identifies short- and long-term goals

- Evaluates as many solutions as possible, emphasizing those that preserve each party's dignity and self-esteem

- Encourages participants to identify one solution, which they agree to try and to evaluate

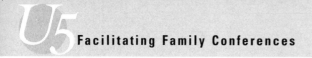

Use Negotiation Strategies to Resolve Conflict

Physicians can use the following negotiation strategies to resolve conflicts:[81]

- Separate people and personalities from the problem
- Clarify the problem
- Brainstorm possible solutions
- Focus on common interests
- Use objective criteria when possible
- Develop solutions that honor both parties

It is important to remember that effective mediation can improve the negotiation process, but it will not resolve underlying, deep-seated conflicts. Due to most patients' limited prognosis when admitted to hospice/palliative programs, physicians need to acknowledge that some family conflicts can be resolved in the time allotted, but others cannot.

When deep-seated conflicts exist, physicians should focus on accomplishing as much as they can, doing as little harm as possible, returning home in the best shape possible, and surviving so they can return to work the next day. Sometimes, in the midst of particularly difficult negotiations, the most therapeutic technique is to leave the room, notice areas of bodily tension, and breathe deeply until some perspective is regained before reentering the fray. Then suggest that negotiations resume after every one has had some time to rethink the issues and can suggest possible solutions.

Denial

Denial and the Patient

Patients usually react to distressing events with characteristic responses formed over the course of a lifetime, e.g., anger, denial, a desire for more information, optimism, acceptance, or certainty that the worst will occur.[2] When patients are faced with news of a life-threatening illness, denial is one of the most common reactions for coping with the implications of approaching death.[82] However, denial is rarely total; it usually waxes and wanes throughout the course of the illness according to the patient's ability to accept the implications of the diagnosis. Most of the time, patients experience several conflicting emotions simultaneously, e.g., denial and anger, fear and hope, or a mix of optimism and despair, all of which are likely to resurface throughout the course of the illness.[2]

A patient's psychological defenses should be respected whenever possible because they are based on life-long patterns of coping with the exigencies of life. Attempts to break down a patient's deep-seated denial are more likely to reflect the needs of caregivers than the actual needs of the patient and should be attempted by psychiatrists only when absolutely necessary. A high degree of denial does present challenges for the team because it:

- Complicates planning for the future

- Often results in underreporting of pain and other distressing symptoms

- Irritates family members and caregivers, which affects their interactions with the patient

Denial and the Family

Often, news of a terminal condition is first disclosed to family members, a situation that may lead to family requests to withhold information from patients.[36] When physicians comply with such requests, they reinforce the mistaken notion that death and dying are too frightening and horrible to discuss, and they exclude patients from participating in healthcare decisions and completing the developmental tasks of the dying.[72] (See *UNIPAC Two: Alleviating Psychological and Spiritual Pain in the Terminally Ill.*) Because a family's request to withhold information about diagnosis and prognosis is likely to reflect its fears and concerns about death, physicians should treat the request with compassion and as an opportunity to:

- Educate family members about the adverse effects of withholding information

- Model effective communication about death-related issues

- Learn about cultural differences regarding communication

Table 8 describes strategies that encourage family/patient communication about dying.

Table 8: Strategies to Encourage Family–Patient Communication about Dying

Normalize Concerns: Acknowledge the difficulty of talking about a serious illness. On a very primitive level, most people believe that death can be prevented by not talking about it—saying the words makes it a reality.

Assess: Gentle but direct questions can elicit additional clues about the family's coping styles and their underlying fears.

- What are some of your concerns about sharing this information with the patient? (Will the family be forced to talk about death every moment of every day until the patient dies? Will the patient's life be miserable every moment of every day until life ends?)
- What is likely to happen if the information is not shared?
- What is the worst thing that is likely to happen if the information is not shared?
- What is likely to happen if the information is shared?
- What is the worst thing that is likely to happen if the information is shared?
- If the worst thing occurs, what is likely to happen next?

Educate: Provide information about the benefits of communicating with patients.

- Most terminally ill patients know that they are dying.
- Studies indicate that most dying patients want more information about their diagnosis and prognosis than anyone realizes.
- Most dying patients want to talk about death-related concerns.
- Withholding information sets a pattern of deception that can destroy a patient's trust in the physician and members of the family.
- Withholding information isolates patients and prevents them from planning for the future and making treatment-related decisions.
- Ethically, physicians cannot refuse to share information with patients.
- Communication is not a one-time event; it is an ongoing process of continued dialog about the patient's life, i.e., joys, struggles, successes, failures, and search for meaning.

If families persist with demands to withhold information, they should be reminded of the following:[62]

- Communication with patients should not stop in the midst of one of the most crucial phases of life.

- Withholding information robs everyone of the possibility of talking about what is happening and results in a painful charade that limits conversation to superficial matters.

- There is no substitute for saying good-by; it is important for the patient and critical for the surviving family.

- Physicians have an ethical obligation to refrain from lying to patients and/or withholding information requested by the patient. However, physicians should also respect family beliefs and cultural differences.

Respect Cultural Differences

Cultural beliefs regarding the sharing of information should be respected.[32] Two brief situations illustrate cultural beliefs regarding communication.

Mr. Hu and His Family. Mr. Hu, an 82-year-old Taiwanese hospice patient with gastric cancer whose symptoms had been well controlled, experienced sudden escalating pain. Mr. Hu rated his pain as 7 on a 10-point scale. The patient's family called the attending physician, a young oncologist new to practice, to request additional medication for pain relief. Before prescribing higher doses, the physician insisted that Mr. Hu give his "consent," which, to the physician, meant that the patient had to acknowledge his imminent death. When the family insisted that the doctor refrain from discussing death with Mr. Hu, the physician refused to prescribe additional medication. Upset, the patient's family called the hospice/palliative care program and requested a change of physicians.

The program's nurse and social worker met with the patient and asked, "Who speaks for you?" Mr. Hu replied, "My family." The hospice medical director notified the attending physician about the family's cultural beliefs regarding communication. The attending physician expressed discomfort with prescribing high doses of opioids and asked the hospice medical director to assume care of the patient.

While examining Mr. Hu, the medical director asked, "Do you know you are quite ill?" The patient nodded. The physician then explained that strong medication was needed to control the pain and asked, "What questions would you like to ask me?" Mr. Hu looked into the doctor's eyes, shook his head, and expressed his gratitude for the physician's visit. During the next few days, the dose of SC hydromorphone had to be rapidly increased to control Mr. Hu's pain, but he died comfortably several days later.

In this case, the attending physician was unfamiliar with the patient's and family's cultural belief that family members should speak for patients and that discussions of death should be avoided. She also was uncomfortable using high doses of a parenteral opioid, probably due to misinformation about the safety of titrated opioids.

The medical director's open-ended question provided Mr. Hu with an opportunity to request more information. Since Mr. Hu declined and had already said that his family made medical decisions for him, the director was not ethically bound to discuss the prognosis.

Native Americans. Several members of an interdisciplinary team gave a presentation on hospice/palliative care to representatives of a Native American tribe. After the team's presentation, the program received no referrals. On follow-up, the program's chaplain met privately with a tribe member and asked for help. The tribe member explained that the presentation was distressing; instead of honoring the tribe's cultural beliefs emphasizing reunion with a cosmic spirit, the presentation focused solely on death. The tribe member suggested that prior to making presentations, the team should:

- Understand the beliefs of different tribes
- Meet with the tribal council and acknowledge the team's ignorance about tribal beliefs
- Ask the council for help structuring the presentation
- Individually tailor the presentation, use appropriate vocabulary, and focus on symptom control instead of death

Confidentiality

In hospice/palliative care settings, patients retain the right to confidentiality. When dying patients and their family members entrust healthcare professionals with their fears, anxiety, remorse, and unfulfilled dreams, they are likely to assume that the information will remain confidential.

Confidentiality is not an absolute obligation—information can be revealed if the patient's condition poses a risk to others—but it should be highly valued.[83] In most cases, concerns arise when a patient shares confidential information with one team member about past events that are now causing psychological or spiritual pain and interfering with the management of physical symptoms. For example, when anxiety, guilt, fear, remorse, or sadness exacerbate physical symptoms that are being treated unsuccessfully with ever-larger dosages of medications, the team member is likely to struggle with the issue of how much to tell to whom. In most cases, patients are willing to negotiate the amount of information shared so that their right to privacy is protected without compromising the team's ability to intervene effectively. Confidentiality is breached when:[36]

- The patient believes information shared with one team member will be kept confidential, **and**
- The patient's information is shared with other team members without the patient's authorization.

Hospice/palliative care programs should develop policies regarding patient confidentiality and the sharing of sensitive information. In the event a patient does not want specific information shared with the rest of the team, balancing the patient's right to privacy with the team's need for information can present ethical dilemmas, particularly when continued secrecy may result in inappropriate treatments.

Example

Charles, a 50-year-old hospice/palliative care patient with lung cancer, is experiencing unrelieved pain, breathlessness, and restlessness. During a visit with the program's chaplain, Charles indicates he is extremely fearful of dying and wants to confide a secret. After being assured of the chaplain's respect for confidentiality, Charles relates that, while serving in Viet Nam, he murdered several civilians and had a child out of wedlock. Now he is very fearful of eternal retribution and is consumed with guilt for the indiscriminate killings, for abandoning the child and mother, and for keeping the child a secret from his wife, Vickie.

The chaplain knows that, in addition to Charles, other people are suffering from Charles's psychological and spiritual distress. The team physician has been treating Charles's restlessness, pain, and dyspnea with ever-larger doses of medication without success and is now questioning her own competence. The social worker is deeply concerned about Charles's obvious but unvoiced emotional distress and is questioning his inability to intervene effectively. Vickie is suffering from an increased sense of isolation from her husband; she wants to comfort Charles but senses that, once again, he is "shutting her out."

During the course of numerous conversations over the next few days, the chaplain reassures Charles that he is a valued and loved human being despite his past failings. The chaplain reminds Charles that other people care about him and tries to negotiate the sharing of some information so that the team can intervene more effectively. Charles agrees to let the chaplain share information about his situation, but only with the physician and only if the actual deeds are not divulged. The chaplain agrees. During the next several weeks, the chaplain encourages Charles to express his love to Vickie. The chaplain also continues to support Charles's search for ways of coming to terms with his entire life.

Special Communications of the Dying Patient

Toward the end of the dying process, some terminally ill patients speak in rambling, disjointed phrases that may indicate either delirium or final communications with very special meanings. Some authors believe that the extraordinary experiences described by dying patients are near-death experiences with special meanings.[84] In their book, *Final Gifts*, Callanan-Pflaum and Kelley recommend educating family members about common themes such as the following, which can help them to decipher any special meanings in the patient's final communications.[85]

- *Being in the presence of the dead*. Terminally ill patients frequently see or talk to someone who has already died.

- *Preparing to travel or change*. Communications about going home, standing in line, or going on a trip may be references to the patient's desire to complete the dying process; they may want permission to die.

- *Seeing a place*. Some dying patients glimpse other worlds or feel as if they are in another place. Usually the dreams or feelings are comforting, but sometimes they create groundless anxieties about mental dysfunction.

- *Choosing when to die*. Some dying patients appear to wait until after they have had a chance to visit with a special family member before dying. On other occasions they may wait until someone has left the room. Very private people may prefer to die while they are alone.

- *Knowing the time of death*. Some terminally ill patients appear to know when they are going to die, even when the usual signs of rapidly approaching death are absent. Patients may call a loved one in the morning to say good-by, seeming to know that death will occur before the next scheduled visit.

Throughout the dying process, caregivers should continue to communicate reassurance and support by:

- Responding in an accepting way to whatever the patient sees or hears

- Asking gentle questions about what the patient is seeing

- Asking patients to repeat statements that aren't understood

- Supporting patients as they die by acknowledging the difficulty of letting go

- Being aware when patients prefer to remain in silence

*Teamwork represents a set of values that encourage[s] listening and construc-
tive response to the views expressed by others, giving others the benefit of the
doubt, providing support, and recognizing the interests and achievements of
others. Such values help teams perform, and they also promote individual performance as well as the performance of an entire organization.*

—Jon Katzenbach and Douglas Smith[86]

*If they don't have scars, they haven't worked on a team. Teams don't just hap-
pen. They slowly and painfully evolve. The process is never complete. The work
involved is usually underestimated.*

—Balfour Mount, MD[87]

Introduction to the Interdisciplinary Approach to Care

Suffering and the Team Approach to Care

Cassell suggests that profound illness is associated with losses affecting all aspects of a patient's life.[88] Significant losses are likely to injure the patient's entire sense of personhood, the complex, interrelated physical, social, emotional, and spiritual dimensions that make up each person. When assaults on personhood are sufficiently injurious, they cause suffering, which Cassell defines as "a state of severe distress associated with events that threaten the intactness of the person."[88]

According to Cassell, "suffering continues until the threat of disintegration has passed or until the integrity of the person can be restored in some other manner."[88] (See *UNIPAC Two: Alleviating Psychological and Spiritual Pain in the Terminally Ill.*)

Because hospice/palliative care focuses not just on relieving physical pain, but also on alleviating suffering experienced by terminally ill patients and their family members, effective interventions require the skills and resources of an entire team of healthcare professionals. The combined professional and personal perspectives of members of an interdisciplinary team are much more likely to meet the complex needs of dying patients and their families.

Medicare Regulations and NHPCO Guidelines

In the United States, the interdisciplinary team approach to caring for dying patients was institutionalized by Medicare, which ties reimbursement to a hospice program's ability to meet basic criteria, among them:[89]

CAAHPM

- Use of an identified interdisciplinary team that includes at least the following core members: a physician, a registered nurse, a social worker, and a pastoral or other counselor

- A specific percentage of hours of volunteer participation

For more information on the Medicare Hospice Benefit, see *UNIPAC One: The Hospice/Palliative Medicine Approach to End-of-Life Care.*

Guidelines developed by the National Hospice and Palliative Care Organization (NHPCO) require team coordination by a qualified healthcare professional to ensure ongoing assessment of the needs of patients and families and implementation of an integrated plan of care.[90]

The Function of the Team

The function of a hospice/palliative care interdisciplinary team is to alleviate the suffering experienced by terminally ill patients and their family members. Each member of the team represents a particular health discipline and uses a discipline-specific framework to explain events and suggest interventions. Ideally, team members pool their expertise to develop an interdisciplinary plan of care addressing the complex needs of each patient and family. The plan must respect the values, beliefs, and goals of individual patients and their families.

Developing an individualized plan of care requires skilled negotiation among team members, patients, and family members. Although healthcare professionals can recommend interventions, patients and family members must implement them, which requires their support of the plan. As the patient's situation changes, the care plan must be revised to meet the patient's needs. The interdisciplinary team approach to care can be time consuming initially, but the resulting multifaceted interventions are more likely to alleviate all contributors to suffering, whether they are physical, emotional, social, or spiritual. The following mnemonic describes the process of developing an individualized plan of care for each patient.

P *Patient's history and life story:* Perform a thorough history that addresses all aspects of total pain, e.g., physical, psychological, social, and spiritual contributors to suffering. Listen carefully to life stories told by patients and family members.

L *Look at objective data:* Obtain needed information from the physical exam and from the patient's self-assessment scales that measure physical pain, depression, or quality of life and consider the need for laboratory work, x-rays, and other information.

A *Assess information:* Assess all information provided by patients, family members, team members, laboratory tests, and self-assessment scales.

N *Negotiate the treatment plan:* Develop an individualized patient care plan with other members of the team. Take into account the patient's values, beliefs, and goals. Negotiate the plan with the patient and family. Revise the plan as needed to better meet the patient's and family's values, beliefs, goals, and changing situation.

The Team and Cost-related Concerns

The Medicare regulations and NHPCO guidelines recognize variations in team composition and frequency of team meetings. Medicare requires participation of only core members in team meetings, but many programs include other healthcare professionals who provide or arrange care for patients and families, e.g., volunteer and bereavement coordinators. Although Medicare regulations require only one team meeting every 2 weeks, in the past many programs reviewed patients at least weekly to address rapid changes in the patients' conditions.

Ideally, each patient and family is evaluated separately by at least the core members of the team. Then the team meets and develops a comprehensive interdisciplinary plan of care. The plan is negotiated with the patient and family until a mutually agreed upon plan is devised. In reality, the process of assessing patients and developing comprehensive plans often falls short of the ideal.

Cost-related concerns affect the frequency and composition of team meetings. Because team meetings fail to generate revenue, some programs now limit the frequency of team meetings to the Medicare minimum. Others include only supervisory staff in team meetings, most of whom have never seen the patients being reviewed. In today's challenging financial climate, it is even more important for team members to:

- Communicate effectively
- Assertively represent their discipline
- Insist that programs meet the physical, social, emotional, and spiritual needs of dying patients and their families

Representing Medicine on the Team

When participating in team meetings, physicians should assertively represent the discipline of medicine while respecting the views of other team members. For example, when deciding whether to initiate heavy sedation to alleviate severe symptoms that cannot be controlled in any other way, most physicians appropriately enlist the help of the entire team. The views of the social worker and chaplain are particularly important because they may shed light on factors contributing to the patient's distress. However, once a decision is made to include sedation as one of several interventions, the physician should decide the type and dose of medication.

The Interdisciplinary Team

Advantages and Disadvantages

Table 9 describes an interdisciplinary team and lists some of its advantages and disadvantages.

Table 9: The Interdisciplinary Team: Description, Advantages, and Disadvantages[91]

Description	Advantages	Disadvantages
■ Involves more than one discipline	■ Integrates many perspectives	■ Initially, decisions take more time
■ Shares information and sets team goals	■ Encourages teamwork to craft creative solutions to difficult problems	■ Members must learn the vocabulary and perspectives of other disciplines
■ Is interdependent, with shared responsibility	■ Develops formal and informal solutions to address complex problems	■ Effort is needed to maintain the team
■ Is structured to encourage collaboration	■ Develops solutions with depth and breadth	■ The team requires time and space to clarify values, renegotiate roles, and resolve conflicts
■ Works on team problems	■ Shares responsibility for leadership	■ Individuals require time to develop leadership skills
■ Shifts leadership, depending on specific issues and areas of expertise	■ Empowers individuals on the team	

Adapted from *Educational Gerontology*, 1996;22(5):437, Drinka TJK, Taylor & Francis: Washington, DC. Reproduced with permission. All rights reserved.

Developmental Phases

Like any other group, interdisciplinary teams undergo a characteristic and sometimes painful developmental process. When faced with crises such as staff cutbacks, mergers, or the loss of key members, even the most effective teams are likely to experience developmental setbacks as they adapt to changed circumstances.[92,93] Table 10 describes the usual developmental phases of an interdisciplinary team.

Table 10: Developmental Phases of an Interdisciplinary Healthcare Team[94]

Phase I: Forming

- Superficial sharing of name and background information
- Members size up and test each other; they categorize each other by outside roles and status
- Members are guarded, more impersonal than personal, a few are active, others are passive
- Uncertainty over purpose exists
- Conflict is neither discussed nor addressed

Phase II: Norming

- Attempt to establish common goals
- Team establishes ground rules and begins to clarify common roles
- Mistrust is exhibited by caution and conformity
- Role overlap becomes evident
- A few members attempt to establish bonds with others who have similar views
- Team may want leader(s) to assume responsibility
- Strategies are used to increase equality of leadership, e.g., rotate leadership
- Defensive communication and disruptive behavior increases
- Frustration exists among team members
- Some members project blame and responsibility toward the perceived leaders
- Competition exists among team members
- Some members come to meetings late or do not attend

Phase III: Confrontation

- Conflicts can no longer be avoided, and some members verbally attack other members
- Increased conflict over leadership, equality, and commitment
- Anxiety over expression of affect
- Some conflicts are addressed in a direct manner
- Some members withdraw from the team
- Search starts for leaders who will resolve conflicts
- Functional leaders emerge
- Realization occurs that power is not equal

(*Continued*)

- Realization occurs that everyone has power for leadership and decision making
- Constructive confrontation results when conflicts occur
- Goals and roles are reclarified
- Coalitions form but change according to team needs

Phase IV: Performing

- Cohesion, high morale
- Differences of members are appreciated
- Members encourage and help each other
- Reality testing increases and grows stronger
- Self-initiated active participation is the norm
- Relationships are strengthened, members trust each other
- Attendance at meetings is regular
- Conflicts seen as normal and are used as impetus for program improvement
- Emphasis is on productivity and problem solving
- Increased responsibility for situation-specific leadership, depending on needed skills

Phase V: Leaving

Individual leaves

- Individual may feel anger toward members of the team in general
- Members deny impending departure because of disbelief and regret
- Team expresses wish for member to remain with the team
- Team may regress to an earlier phase
- Individual may express happiness over leaving the team

Team terminates

- Some members withdraw; depression and sadness result
- Expressions of team's superiority are made
- Feelings are expressed as testimonials
- Team membership is affirmed as a valuable experience

Characteristics of Effective Teams

Interdisciplinary teams perform two separate functions: task functions (what the team does) and maintenance functions (how the team members interact).[95] In general, effective teams:

- Agree on a common set of principles, goals, and measurable objectives[86]
- Expect members to represent their discipline's current practice standards and share responsibility for team functioning[92]
- Provide training in team interaction, leadership, communication, and conflict resolution[95]

Table 11 summarizes the characteristics of effective interdisciplinary teams; they are covered in more detail in the remainder of this section.

Institutional Support

Effective interdisciplinary teams are essential for providing hospice/palliative care, but they do not just happen. They require institutional support and commitment to:

- Hire knowledgeable professionals with strong skills in communication and problem solving who will assertively represent their discipline's unique body of knowledge[95]

Table 11: Characteristics of Effective Interdisciplinary Teams[80,86,92,95–97]

- Institutional support
- Shared philosophy, goals, and norms; goal directed
- Effective leaders and leadership styles, with emphasis on coordination
- Emphasis on team interdependency, with role recognition and support
- Skilled communication and problem solving, especially when difficulties arise
- Shared decision making
- Flexibility and openness to new ideas
- Documentation of care that ensures accountability and confidentiality
- Effective collaboration with other healthcare providers, teams, and organizations
- Formal team self-evaluation to improve future performance
- Synergy, camaraderie, empowerment, and fun

- Support continuing education and training related to professional skills *and* team functioning

- Provide adequate organizational resources to support the team: room, administrative staff support, and time to fulfill the basic functions of the team, including regular meetings to exchange information and plan comprehensive interventions

- Support regularly scheduled team evaluations and self-assessments to determine the team's effectiveness in terms of task *and* function. Evaluations and self-assessments should address the roles of the administrative staff, the management team, the interdisciplinary team as a whole, and individual members of the care team.

A smoothly functioning interdisciplinary team is vital for effective patient care. However, the primary goal of hospice/palliative care teams is alleviating the patient's and family's suffering, not maintaining the team. Adequate administrative support should be provided to establish and maintain a qualified, well-trained interdisciplinary team of healthcare professionals to provide needed care. Then all team members, including physicians, must encourage careful allocation of resources to provide comprehensive, high-quality care for patients and families.

NOTE: Executives and managers may intentionally minimize the amount of time that they spend together, but members of teams need to be given enough time to learn to work together as a team.[86]

Shared Principles, Goals, Objectives, and Norms

Depending on their size and maturity, hospice/palliative care programs are likely to use at least two types of teams: a management team and one or more interdisciplinary care teams. Regardless of a team's specific function, its members must agree on the team's guiding principles and its purpose or reason for existence, goals, and objectives for achieving these goals.

- Members of effective teams spend significant time and effort defining principles, purposes, and goals to which they subscribe both collectively and individually.[86] The principles, purposes, and many of the goals of hospice/palliative care interdisciplinary teams are predetermined by the nature of the work. For example, members of interdisciplinary hospice/palliative care teams must be committed to symptom control, relief of suffering, an interdisciplinary team approach to whole-person care, and honest and compassionate communication. Other goals may include educating medical students and serving specific populations, such as children or patients with AIDS.

Effective teams translate their purpose and goals into realistic, specific, measurable outcome objectives that they use to evaluate their effectiveness. Examples of measurable outcome objectives include:

- Physical pain and other symptoms are reduced to acceptable levels within a specific number of hours or days.

- The patient's and family's existential pain is reduced to acceptable levels within a specific number of days, weeks, or months.

- The patient is receiving all needed financial and other resources from governmental and community programs within a specific number of days or weeks.

Specific, measurable outcome objectives serve as powerful contributors to performance, job satisfaction, and an enhanced sense of purpose and meaning. Specific goals support clear communication, constructive conflict, and goal-directed care and are more likely to result in effective interventions. Measurable goals also provide tools for determining the effectiveness of a team's individual and collective interventions.

Norms are unwritten rules that govern a group's behavior, i.e., what is acceptable or unacceptable.[80,98] In most groups, norms are unspoken, unexamined, and often confusing for new team members. Because group norms influence every aspect of team functioning, open discussion can clarify the group's rules and improve team functioning.

- Is conflict dealt with openly and honestly or is it hidden or ignored?

- Is discussion of certain subjects prohibited?

- Are team members allowed to express only certain kinds of feelings?

- Do all team members actively participate in team meetings, or just a few? What does nonparticipation indicate in terms of honoring the specialized knowledge and expertise of each team member?

- Are people who work with dying patients allowed to set limits on their involvement to achieve a balanced life or must they put patient care ahead of all other priorities, including interaction with their own families?

Effective Leaders and Leadership Styles with Emphasis on Coordination

In healthcare settings, physicians often serve as leaders of *multidisciplinary* teams. When serving on *interdisciplinary* teams, physicians participate as colleagues, and leadership is shared depending on the needs of specific situations.[92] Nevertheless, the patient's attending physician is medically and legally responsible for the patient's medical care, and the hospice medical director is ultimately responsible for the program's medical care of all patients.

In hospice/palliative care settings the terms *leader* and *coordinator* are administrative labels that do not necessarily imply higher status or the right to make unilateral decisions.[92] For example, in many mature programs the designated team leader is likely to be a healthcare professional with strong organizational and facilitation skills. Regardless of who is appointed, effective team leaders exhibit the skills listed in Table 12.

Table 12: Skills of Effective Leaders[80,95]

- Plan and facilitate meetings with clear objectives and stay on track.
- Encourage use of a problem-solving approach.
- Encourage comprehensive interventions that meet the needs of patients and families.
- Ensure effective coordination and communication.
- Share team decisions with necessary parties.
- Keep extraneous anecdotal information to a minimum.
- Help motivate other team members to the highest possible standards of care.
- Adapt leadership style to specific circumstances.
- Balance problem-solving and task-oriented behavior with nurturing and motivating.
- Encourage regularly scheduled self-evaluations to measure the team's effectiveness in terms of its internal functioning and its ability to alleviate suffering.

Effective interdisciplinary teams share leadership. For example, a physician and a social worker may share leadership during a patient–family conference, with the physician leading a discussion of distressing physical symptoms and the social worker leading discussions of the patient's and/or family's adjustment difficulties. Physicians are expected to provide leadership when the team is developing the medical component of a patient's care plan.

Effective leaders adapt their leadership styles to the needs of specific groups or situations. For example, a more autocratic, directive style might be appropriate for teams new to hospice/palliative care, but a democratic style is likely to be more effective for teams of seasoned hospice/palliative care professionals. Common leadership styles, each of which can be effective in specific situations, include:

- *Autocratic:* Group members may have input, but the leader makes the final decision.
- *Oligarchic:* A small, specialized group makes final decisions.
- *Democratic:* Group members participate equally in decision making.
- *Laissez-faire:* Group members make their own decisions and go their own way.

Emphasis on Team Interdependency with Role Recognition and Support

Members of effective teams recognize that their ability to alleviate a patient's or family's suffering depends on the collective ability of the team. However, they also recognize the importance of individual responsibility and accountability. Effective teams:

- Recognize, honor, and utilize the expertise of each member of the team

- Carefully evaluate how each discipline can contribute to the team's overall goals

- Recognize the need for role definition and role flexibility

- Expect team members to represent their discipline's current practice standards and to participate fully in team meetings

- Expect team and individual accountability for developing interventions and implementing agreed-upon interventions

- Understand that a team's success depends on each member's ability to communicate effectively, work both independently and interdependently, and recognize individual and collective responsibilities

- Provide support and ongoing training to maximize the team's effectiveness and the professional growth of each team member

Role recognition and support are important components of interdisciplinary teamwork. For example, chaplains are not expected to become the team expert on assessing and managing neuropathic or bone pain, but they should be able to recognize obvious signs of uncontrolled physical pain, ask patients if they are in pain, and report uncontrolled pain to appropriate staff. Physicians are not expected to become experts on assessing and alleviating spiritual pain, but they should be able to complete a preliminary assessment of spiritual pain as part of an overall history and discuss basic spiritual questions when appropriate.

Role flexibility is essential when caring for dying patients and their families. Nurses and home health aides often provide basic supportive counseling for distressed patients and family members during home visits. And social workers and chaplains may need to help patients to the bathroom, straighten their sheets, or help them to find more comfortable positions.

Role-related difficulties that affect performance and contribute to stress include role ambiguity, role conflict, and role overload.[80,98]

Role Ambiguity. Role ambiguity occurs when healthcare professionals are uncertain how to participate on interdisciplinary teams, when little or no orientation is provided, and when team members are expected to perform roles for which they have little or no education or training. Teams can reduce role ambiguity by discussing the roles of team

---

member, listing all the tasks associated with each role, and outlining areas of role uniqueness and overlap.[92] Role ambiguity is most likely to occur when:

- Traditional roles must be adapted to nontraditional settings.[80]
- Roles and expectations are poorly defined or not clearly communicated.
- Priorities are not clearly communicated.
- Tasks are not clearly defined.

Role Conflict. *Interrole conflict.* Differing professional perspectives enhance the team's ability to provide comprehensive interventions. They also inevitably lead to periodic role conflicts among team members about which is the best intervention. When interrole conflicts are handled effectively, differences of opinion often result in interventions that better meet the patient's and family's physical, social, emotional, and spiritual needs. Differences of opinion also provide team members with a better understanding of each discipline's perspective. However, unresolved, ongoing differences can lead to serious conflicts, which are more likely to occur when:[80]

- Team members believe that their contributions are consistently overlooked.
- Team members believe that their specific discipline serves a special patient advocacy role not shared by other disciplines.

Problem-based rather than personality-based discussions of patient–family problems can reduce the number of role conflicts. See "Conflict Resolution" on page 87.

Intrarole conflict. In addition to interrole conflicts among team members, team members are likely to experience intrarole conflict. For example, the program's medical director is expected to provide expert symptom management *and* report to executive directors, boards, and, in the case of for-profit programs, to owners and investors, all of whom are concerned with the program's financial health and, in some cases, with profit sharing. When programs are reluctant to cover the costs of the expensive palliative treatments sometimes needed to control difficult symptoms, the medical director may experience intrarole conflict. The "physician" wants to provide the most effective intervention regardless of cost, but the "medical administrator" wants to protect the program's financial health. On occasion, a medical director's insistence on providing needed but costly treatments or on maintaining low patient–staff ratios results in strained relationships with the program's administrators, owners, and investors.

Role Overload. Role overload most often occurs when team members:

- Are expected to complete an unrealistic amount of work in a given time frame
- Are expected to take on more responsibility without additional training or support

- Have unrealistic personal expectations concerning their own productivity

- Experience crises in their personal lives that result in additional role demands

Communication and Problem-solving Skills

Teams depend on professional expertise, communication, and problem-solving skills to achieve their goals. Clear communication is essential; it provides the foundation on which rests the team's ability to function. Effective communication:[48,99]

- Enhances coordination

- Facilitates the exchange of needed information

- Advances the team's goals

- Helps to break down barriers

- Improves understanding

- Confirms and supports team members

- Encourages ethical analysis

- Respects everyone in the group

- Helps listeners to keep an open mind

- Avoids profanity, sexism, and stereotypes

On effective teams, team members feel free to speak candidly and participate fully in team discussions. They also:[100]

- Allow others to speak

- Respect the opinions of other team members

- Recognize the importance of thoroughly discussing each patient's situation (within reasonable time frames)

- Examine the burdens and benefits of suggested interventions

Shared Decision Making

Interdisciplinary teams rely on shared decision making. However, rapid changes in a patient's condition and acute patient or family needs may require immediate decisions by one or two members of the team. Emergency decisions are discussed later with the entire team. When groups of people make decisions, they generally use one or more of the methods listed in Table 13.

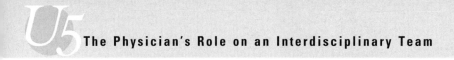

Table 13: Methods of Decision Making

Default: No decision is made (which is itself a decision). No one cares enough to voice an opinion, or team members are reluctant to voice an opinion because it is not politically expedient or because it conflicts with spoken or unspoken group norms.

Unilateral: The most powerful person on the team (sometimes the team leader) makes the final decision.

Oligarchic: Decisions are made by a small group, who may reverse or alter decisions made during the team meeting.

Majority Rule: Members of the team vote and the majority wins, even if the decision is not in the best interests of the patient, family, or program. Prior to voting, team members should decide on the majority percentage (e.g., 51% or 75%).

Unanimity: All members agree (or appear to agree) with a certain line of action.

Consensus: Discussion continues until all members reach a compromise, even though no one may be completely satisfied with the final decision.

Openness to New Ideas

Members of effective teams understand that continuing education and openness to new ideas and perspectives are essential components of improved team performance and professional competence.

Effective Collaboration with Other Healthcare Providers, Teams, and Organizations

Effective collaboration with other patient care organizations, such as nursing facilities, hospitals, and home healthcare agencies, identifies common goals and interests, reduces professional isolation, and improves patient care.

Formal Team Self-evaluation

Like any other group or system, hospice/palliative care teams eventually develop lives of their own and begin to protect their own existence. To ensure the team's continued focus on alleviating patient–family distress, effective teams schedule regular self-assessments focusing on realistic goal attainment and team functioning. They examine questions such as the following: Are the team's expectations realistic? Do interventions effectively alleviate the patient's and family's physical, spiritual, emotional, and social pain? How does the team measure its effectiveness? Are outcome measures used to determine progress toward specific goals? Is the team operating in the most efficient manner? Are all disciplines represented and accountable? Are roles as clearly defined as possible? Is the team receiving adequate institutional support? Do all team members have access to continuing education? Is the team developing dysfunctional behavioral patterns such as avoiding conflict at all costs, becoming professionally isolated, or spending more time on team maintenance than on patient and family care?

Synergy, Camaraderie, Empowerment, and Fun

Effective teams are characterized by good morale, support, and encouragement that helps to relieve the inevitable stresses associated with caring for patients who are terminally ill. Members of effective teams:[96]

- Support each other and temporarily lighten the load of team members who are experiencing personal difficulties or work-related stress

- Realize that no one member is indispensable, which allows team members to leave at the end of the day, confident that others will care for patients during their absence

- Recognize the importance of positive feedback and recognition to promote team performance

- Recognize the importance of professional and personal growth and appropriate humor (see "Use Appropriate Humor" on pages 37–39)

Barriers to Effective Teamwork

Table 14 describes common problems and barriers to effective teamwork.

Signs and Symptoms of Dysfunctional Teams

All groups operate in ways that support or impede a group's identified goals. Even functional groups often become temporarily dysfunctional when stressors occur: the assimilation of new team members; the resignation, death, or dismissal of important group members; changes in funding; or dysfunctional behavior on the part of an important group member. Symptoms of dysfunctional team behavior may be difficult to assess due to:

- Denial, or the reluctance to admit that the team is becoming dysfunctional

- Helplessness, or uncertainty about how to intervene

- Unawareness, or lack of awareness of the symptoms of dysfunctional team behavior

Early recognition of the symptoms of dysfunctional team behavior increases the likelihood that effective interventions will return the team to healthy functioning. Table 15 describes selected symptoms of dysfunctional teams, many of which were adapted from White's "dynamics of organizational incest."[41]

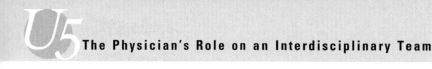

Table 14: Common Problems and Barriers to Effective Teamwork[96,100]

Breakdown in Eliciting Information. Teams need to gather enough information to make good decisions about treatment. When team leaders use only closed questions or brief assertions, it is unlikely that other team members will provide enough information to make good decisions. Examples: "Did you order that? Do you want the patient to think we don't care?"

Promotional Leadership. Promotional leadership occurs when team leaders or powerful team members voice an idea or opinion before asking for team input; this affects the candor of the team and usually occurs unintentionally, but it can be used in a subtle way to prevent or limit discussion while appearing to be open-minded. Example: "I think we should transfer this patient back home immediately. Now I'd like to hear what you think."

Private Agendas. Periodic conflict is expected because effective teams are candid and often debate the best interventions to use in specific situations. Effective team members "tell it like it is" and sometimes argue. They are not always cautious, nor do they make safe, innocuous comments or suggestions. However, when private agendas develop and cliques occur, candor disappears, asking for information becomes a method for demeaning team members, and one-upmanship replaces teamwork.

Insufficient Alternatives. Failure to explore all options before making decisions can prematurely close discussion and result in the team's wishing that they had spent more time discussing alternatives before taking action. Although exploring alternatives is time consuming, it generally results in better ideas and decisions.

Lack of Candor. Good decisions are based on complete information, which requires accurate disclosure of relevant information by all team members. Barriers to candor include personal reasons for not being honest (not wanting to hurt someone's feelings or put someone on the spot) and team politics (team members may distort information because it is the expedient thing to do). Challenges to the team's values, norms, goals, and objectives should be honored.

Lack of Ongoing Self-assessment. Lack of careful analysis of the team's functioning and effectiveness can lead to scapegoating, i.e., an unpopular person is viewed as causing all the team's problems. Regularly scheduled self-assessments should address the team's strengths, weaknesses, and functioning.

Lack of Responsibility. The emphasis on collective team responsibility and shared leadership can result in lack of individual accountability and ineffective leadership. Overdependency on team members leads to a loss of personal responsibility, accountability, and independence.

Unresolved Conflict. Ongoing disagreements about policies often generate conflict; e.g., assigned tasks cannot be completed within usual working hours. When constant self-sacrifice is required, the program's structure and staffing should be examined. Good patient care should not depend on the team's ongoing willingness to devalue other aspects of their lives, such as marital and family relationships, spiritual and religious growth, and self-care activities.

Failure to Communicate Team Decisions to Others. Even when excellent plans are generated, they are unlikely to succeed unless all parties are willing to collaborate. Team decisions must be effectively communicated to those who implement plans, e.g., home health aides, volunteers, and home care nurses.

Table 15: Symptoms of a Dysfunctional Team[41]

Closed Versus Open Structure

- Closed structure is likely when team members think of themselves as "us" and everyone else as "them." Members of closed teams are fearful of people who want to attend team meetings, but are not viewed as members of the "official" team; for example, a patient's family member or minister, or a nursing home or hospital staff person who cares for the patient and wants to attend the team review of that patient.

Team Leader Becomes Dysfunctional

- In the long run, "one-person" interdisciplinary teams that rely on the skills of a charismatic team member are ineffective. The following behaviors are characteristic of dysfunctional leadership behavior: the leader does not allow questions about decisions, takes credit for all the program's success and blames others for its failures, schedules team meetings at times that exclude certain members such as attending physicians, and forms inappropriate relationships with certain team members.

Team or Program Isolation from the Rest of the Healthcare Community

- Collaboration with other healthcare providers is limited or nonexistent, team members are suspicious of other healthcare providers, access to outside professional organizations is limited, professional travel is restricted to a few favored members of the team.

- Team members socialize exclusively with one another and believe that only they understand the stresses of working with dying patients. Team members believe that the special nature of working with terminally ill patients absolves them from professional ethical guidelines and/or from emotional presence in other relationships, e.g., marital or parental roles.

Self-perpetuation and Homogenization of Members or Staff

- Team members are recruited only from within the team's social network.

Isolation and Scapegoating of Unpopular Team Members

- Team members who question policies, decisions, or group norms are isolated.

All Problems Projected onto a Common Outside Enemy

- Blame for all the team's problems is projected onto funding sources, other healthcare organizations, computer systems, unpopular managers, or members of the community.

Increased Interpersonal Conflict

- Unresolved conflicts lead to passive aggressive behavior instead of conflict resolution, gossip instead of direct communication, and increased turnover as members who are unwilling to work in a dysfunctional setting leave for other positions.

Absenteeism

- Frequent absences indicate that team meetings are no longer meeting the needs of team members.

(Continued)

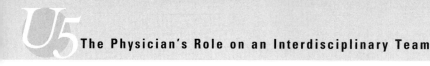

Outsourcing of Care

- Frequent outsourcing of care and overuse of inpatient care can be a sign of inadequate training or lack of time to provide effective care, e.g., all anxious or depressed patients are immediately referred to a psychiatrist.

Focus Shifts from Patient Care to the Team's Personal and Interpersonal Problems

- As team dysfunction increases, meetings consume much of the work week, and energy is directed to resolving conflicts, providing team support, and maintaining the team.

- Patient care is not adequately addressed because the team's energy is being expended on its own problems.

Development of Problematic Social and Sexual Relationships between Team Members or Team Members and Patients

- Inappropriate social and sexual relationships are indicators of serious dysfunction.

Managing Team Conflict

Interpersonal Conflict Resolution Skills

Ajemian describes the following problem-solving approach for managing interpersonal team conflict.[80] During the discussion it is important for both parties to protect the self-respect of the other person and to work together to develop possible solutions.

- *Timing.* As soon as emotions have cooled, deal with the problem instead of waiting.

- *Location.* Meet in a private area, free from interruptions.

- Describe what happened. "I was not told that my patient, Mrs. Smith, died over the weekend."

- Describe the emotional consequences. "On Monday morning, I was embarrassed when I went to Mrs. Smith's house for a home visit. Her husband told me she was dead and said I should know more about my patients."

- Specify what you want to happen in the future and how you can help. "I think home care nurses should be better informed about weekend events."

- Describe the consequences if behavior is changed. "There will be better communication and less confusion on Monday mornings."

- Together generate possible solutions. "We could work with a small group of involved parties and draft a procedure for communicating weekend events."

- Choose an agreed-upon solution.
- Form a plan, try it for a while, and evaluate the effectiveness of the intervention.

Skills for Facilitating Conflict Resolution

When conflicts cannot be resolved by involved parties and outside intervention is required, third-party facilitators should use conflict resolution skills, such as those described by Ajemian:[80]

- Welcome the existence of conflict, bring it into the open, and use it as the basis for positive change.
- Clarify the nature of the problem—is this the real problem?
- Reduce the areas of conflict. List specific problems and confine the discussion to problems identified by both parties.
- Suggest procedures and ground rules.
- Identify short- and long-term goals.
- Identify factors that keep the individuals in conflict.
- Suggest and then evaluate as many solutions as possible, looking for those that preserve each party's dignity and self-esteem.
- Agree on one solution, record it, and ensure that both parties agree on the meaning of the solution as it is written.
- Try the solution and then reevaluate it.

Members of an Interdisciplinary Team: Roles and Functions

Characteristics of Effective Team Members

Table 16 lists several characteristics of effective interdisciplinary team members as described by Ajemian.

The Core Team

Medicare regulations require the involvement of at least four core team members who develop and implement the patient's initial plan of care and review it at least every 2 weeks:

- Physician
- Registered nurse

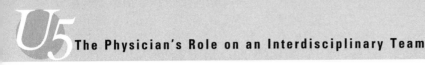

Table 16: Characteristics of Effective Team Members[80]

- Professional competence
- Knowledge of their discipline; they represent the most current knowledge and skills of their profession
- Previous work experience within their discipline
- Willingness to work on common goals and subordinate personal agendas for the good of the patient and family
- Ability to work together to identify problems and develop team goals
- Willingness to trust others
- Patience, flexibility, openness, and tolerance of ambiguity
- Professional and personal maturity; ability to accept oneself, set personal limits, and take responsibility for actions and behavior
- Effective communication with other members of the team
- Respect for others and their contributions; respect for the role of each team member
- Willingness to support colleagues and provide validation, recognition, and encouragement
- Appropriate use of humor
- Support of continuing quality improvement

- Social worker
- Pastoral or other counselor

Because spiritual support is an integral component of end-of-life care, most programs employ a chaplain to serve as the core counselor. The composition of extended teams depends on the program's resources and the needs of patients and their families. Some programs employ other counselors with special expertise in children's grief or family counseling. Many programs include the volunteer and bereavement coordinators. Specialized team members include pharmacists and physical, speech, occupational, art, and music therapists.

Patients and family members are considered members of the team, but they rarely attend team meetings. In most cases, team members report the patient's and family's concerns during team meetings and request suggested interventions. Team members then meet with patients and family members, discuss suggested interventions, and develop mutually agreed-upon plans of action.

To help physicians to understand the roles of various team members, the following sections describe the roles and functions of physicians, nurses, social workers, counselors, and volunteer and bereavement coordinators.

Physicians

Table 17 describes common roles and functions of physicians associated with hospice/palliative care programs. Smaller programs generally employ one physician, who serves as a part- or full-time medical director. Larger programs often employ a full-time medical director and sometimes one or more team physicians, whose specific functions depend on the program's needs. The medical director or team physician may serve as a patient's attending physician.

Table 17: Roles and Functions of Physicians[90,102,104]

Attending Physician

- Provide admitting diagnosis and prognosis
- Provide current medical findings
- Remain actively involved in the patient's care or transfer care to a hospice physician
- Work closely with other members of the IDT
- Order medications and treatments
- Make inpatient and home visits as needed
- Participate in family conferences
- Provide medical management of conditions unrelated to the terminal illness
- Designate an emergency on-call physician
- Ask for a consultation from the hospice medical director or palliative care team physician when distressing symptoms persist

Hospice Medical Director

- Assume overall responsibility for the medical component of a hospice patient's care
- Confirm terminal prognosis and provide a second-physician certification for Medicare or Medicaid eligibility
- Recertify patients as terminally ill at Medicare or Medicaid-required intervals
- Determine medical appropriateness of treatment options and goals
- Consult with referring or attending physicians
- Evaluate patients in home or inpatient settings
- Prescribe treatments and medications as approved by referring physicians
- Serve as patient's referring or attending physician when requested or necessary
- Actively participate in IDT meetings and provide medical guidance for care plans

(*Continued*)

- Provide consultation and problem solving to IDT
- Educate team members, other healthcare professionals, patients and families, and lay public about the hospice/palliative approach to caring for terminally ill patients
- Direct and participate in quality assurance activities and research to improve patient care
- Provide medical administration according to program policies
- Act as community advocate for hospice/palliative care

Hospice/Palliative Care Team Physician

- Fulfill many of the same functions as the medical director, generally with more emphasis on patient care and less on administration
- Ensure that all patients cared for by the team receive needed services and appropriate palliative medical care
- Actively participate in team meetings
- Visit patients in home and inpatient settings

Provisions in the 1997 Budget Reconciliation Bill allow hospice programs to contract for physician services with independent physicians or physician groups. In most cases, the patient's attending physician continues to serve in that capacity after the patient is admitted for hospice/palliative care.

In addition to the physician's roles listed in Table 17, hospice/palliative care programs arrange for consultant physicians when needed to ensure that patients receive care consistent with the principles of palliative medicine.[101,102] Examples include radiation therapy for palliative treatment of bone metastases provided by a radiation therapist, immobilization of pathological fractures by an orthopedist, and therapeutic thoracentesis by a pulmonologist.[103]

The medical director of a Medicare-certified hospice program is responsible for the medical components of the Plans of Care of all hospice patients electing the Medicare Hospice Benefit. If the medical director is not assuming overall responsibility, the program is not in compliance with required conditions of participation. The medical director or the physician member of the interdisciplinary team also is responsible for:

- Certifying and recertifying that a patient is terminally ill
- Participating with the team to establish patient-specific plans of care
- Routinely reviewing and updating plans of care to ensure that patients and families are receiving needed care and services
- Collaborating with the patient's attending physician.

Hospice/palliative care emphasizes the palliation of complex, rapidly changing symptoms. Recently, cost-related concerns have led to reductions in physician involvement with patient care and reliance on treatment protocols. Instead of less physician involvement, effective symptom management is most often associated with increased involvement by physicians with specialized training in pain and symptom management.

Board Certification in Hospice/Palliative Medicine

Board certification in hospice/palliative medicine is recommended for physicians caring for terminally ill patients, in particular for physicians associated with hospice/palliative care programs. In the United States, the American Board of Hospice and Palliative Medicine developed the first national physician certification examination in hospice/palliative medicine. Information on board certification is available from the American Board of Hospice and Palliative Medicine at www.abhpm.org.

Criteria to take the examination include:

- Current licensure as a physician in the Unites States, or equivalent in other countries
- Certification by a board approved by the American Board of Medical Specialties, or the equivalent in other countries
- At least 2 years of experience in the clinical practice of medicine following residency
- At least 2 years of experience working as a member of an interdisciplinary team
- Direct participation in the active care of at least 50 terminally ill patients in the preceding 3 years

Table 18 lists general qualifications for physicians associated with hospice/palliative care programs.

Nurses

Registered nurses working in hospice/palliative care settings should have experience in physical assessment, pain and symptom management, and home care. Licensed practical nurses may serve as primary care nurses as long as they are supervised by a registered nurse.

Hospice/palliative care settings usually offer more opportunities for leadership, participation in decision making, and involvement with assessing and alleviating a patient's physical symptoms and the patient's and family's emotional, spiritual, and social distress. Table 19 describes several roles and functions of hospice/palliative care nurses. The Hospice Palliative Nurses Association (formerly the Hospice Nurses Association)

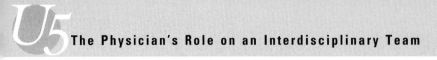

Table 18: Qualifications of Hospice/Palliative Care Physicians[90,104]

Hospice/Palliative Care Medical Director

- Doctor of medicine or osteopathy with current license to practice and prescribe scheduled drugs
- Staff privileges at participating healthcare facilities
- Working knowledge of common terminal illnesses
- Expertise in applying the principles of hospice/palliative care
- Expertise in palliation of common symptoms of terminal illnesses
- Administrative expertise
- Competence in communicating with patient, family, and team members
- Ability to collaborate effectively with other members of the IDT
- Skill in consultation and liaison relationships with other heathcare professionals
- Ability to teach healthcare professionals and lay public
- Ability to participate in research protocols as appropriate
- A deep concern for the plight of dying patients

Hospice/Palliative Care Team Physician

- Identical to those for medical directors, with the exception of administrative expertise

Attending Physician

- Doctor of medicine or osteopathy with current license to practice and prescribe scheduled drugs
- Familiarity with the principles and practice of hospice/palliative care
- Willingness to learn more about palliative management of common symptoms
- Ability to work closely with the IDT

---

formed the National Board for Certification of Hospice Palliative Nurses, which developed the first national certification examination for hospice nurses. Successful candidates earn the credential CRNH (Certified Registered Nurse Hospice). For more information, go to www.hpna.org.

Social Workers

In hospice/palliative care, psychosocial assessments focus on the patient's and family's:

- Understanding of the diagnosis and prognosis

Table 19: Roles and Functions of Hospice Nurses[90,104]

Common Roles

- Patient care coordinator
- Primary care nurse
- Assessment or admission nurse
- On-call nurse

Functions

- Perform physical assessments
- Perform preliminary assessments of the patient's and family's emotional, social, spiritual, and environmental needs
- Coordinate care so that patients or family members receive needed:
  Supplies, e.g., durable medical equipment, diapers, bedside commodes
  Treatments, e.g., medications, physiotherapy
  Interventions to alleviate physical, psychological, social, and spiritual pain
- Provide direct patient care
- Educate patients and families, other healthcare professionals, and volunteers
- Supervise licensed nurses, home heath aides, and homemakers
- Communicate with team members, including attending physicians, the hospice medical director, team physicians
- Assist patients and families with identifying needs
- Provide support at the time of death
- Document problems, appropriate goals, interventions, and patient and family responses
- Participate in IDT meetings and prepare the plan of care

- Strengths and available resources
- Problems precipitated by the terminal illness
- Past experiences of loss and how they were handled
- Unique cultural and social factors affecting the patient's and family's beliefs about illness and health care
- Expectations and plans for the future

CAAHPM

Although team members often think of social workers as providing only instrumental services (those related to community liaison and referral),[80] social workers with advanced degrees and certifications often are qualified to provide counseling services, including short-term therapy for death-related issues. Social workers also may function as bereavement counselors and/or bereavement coordinators. Table 20 lists common social work roles and functions in hospice/palliative care programs. Ideally, hospice social workers have earned a master's degree, with clinical experience appropriate to the counseling and casework needs of terminally ill patients and their family members.

Counselors, Chaplains, and Bereavement Counselors

Medicare regulations require that a pastoral or other counselor serve as the fourth member of the core team. Because spiritual pain is such a frequent contributor to suffering,

---

Table 20: Roles and Functions of Social Workers[90,104]

Instrumental Services

- Prepare comprehensive psychosocial assessments
- Identify needed community resources
- Make referrals to community resources and provide liaison functions when needed
- Participate in discharge planning
- Act as a liaison with community groups
- Provide patient and family education about finances, advance directives, and psychosocial issues
- Educate patients and families, other healthcare professionals, and volunteers
- Communicate with team members, including attending physicians, the hospice medical director, and team physicians
- Assist patients and families with identifying needs
- Document problems, appropriate goals, interventions, and patient and family responses
- Participate in IDT meetings and prepare the plan of care

Counseling

- Provide emotional support for patients and family members
- Provide individual counseling for patients and family members
- Provide family counseling
- Provide bereavement counseling

---

most hospice programs fulfill the Medicare counseling requirement with a chaplain who provides or coordinates the provision of spiritual services. Large programs may also employ other counselors who, depending on their education, training, and areas of expertise, provide additional services, such as short-term psychotherapy and bereavement counseling. Table 21 describes the roles and functions of the various counselors often associated with hospice/palliative care.

Table 21: Roles and Functions of Counselors, Chaplains, and Bereavement Counselors[90,104]

Chaplain

- Prepare comprehensive spiritual assessments of each patient and family that identify religious and spiritual strengths, needs, and resources

- Coordinate, arrange for, or provide religious and spiritual care in keeping with the patient's and family's belief system

- Provide pastoral care and support and facilitate the patient's or family's search for hope and meaning

- Provide pastoral counseling related to death and the afterlife, guilt, fear, loss, and existential concerns

- Refer patients and families to appropriate religious or spiritual leaders on request

- Act as a liaison with local religious and spiritual leaders

- Coordinate and collaborate with local clergy, other counselors, and organized religious bodies to meet the spiritual and religious needs of terminally ill patients

- Develop and facilitate educational programs for healthcare professionals, volunteers, lay public, and local religious and spiritual organizations and leaders on spiritual issues related to death and dying

Grief or Bereavement Counselor

- Assist team with identification of individual at risk for complicated bereavement

- Prepare comprehensive bereavement assessments for individuals at risk

- Develop bereavement assessment tools, interventions, and referral sources

- Provide bereavement support for families for at least 12 months after the patient's death

- Provide bereavement counseling or referrals to other specialists, such as psychiatrists or therapists, when needed

- Develop and facilitate bereavement support groups

- Coordinate and facilitate memorial services for bereaved families

- Work within and contribute to an IDT

- Educate health professionals, volunteers, and lay public about bereavement issues related to death and dying

Table 22: Functions and Qualifications of Volunteers[90,106]

Functions Include:

- Patient care

- Patient companionship while family members rest, run errands, etc.

- Patient and family support: errands, cooking, sitting, light housework, yard work, home repair.

- Bereavement support and follow-up

- Pastoral support

- Lay public education about hospice concepts of care

- Assisting with music and art therapy

- Administrative support

- Fund raising

- Consultant help with legal advice, accounting, computers, and brochure design

Qualifications Include:

- Completion of a comprehensive volunteer training program

- Completion of advanced volunteer training for specific areas

- Emotional maturity, nonjudgmental attitude

- Good communication and listening skills

- Commitment to the philosophy and goals of hospice/palliative care

- Discretion and respect for confidentiality

- Sense of self-worth and empathy

- Willingness to make a commitment

- Resolution of personal losses or serve only in administrative roles

- Freedom from need to promote special religious or work views, life-styles, or other personal missions

- Compassion and sensitive care regardless of a patient's or family member's race, creed, sexual orientation, and religious or political beliefs

- Ability to recognize volunteer limits, accept supervision, and follow volunteer policies and procedures

Volunteers and the Volunteer Coordinator

Hospice is the only Medicare-funded program that mandates volunteer participation.[105] Medicare-certified hospice programs must provide specific types of volunteer training and must deliver a specific percentage of hours of volunteer participation. (For more information about the Medicare Hospice Benefit, see *UNIPAC One: The Hospice/Palliative Medicine Approach to Caring for the Terminally Ill.*) Many of the functions and qualifications of hospice volunteers are described in Table 22. Volunteers are considered members of the team and, after being reminded of the importance of patient confidentiality, can attend team meetings during reviews of the patients they care for.

Volunteer coordinators with demonstrated abilities and experience in communication, management, and organizational skills are responsible for the recruitment, selection, training, supervision and retention of volunteers. Many of the functions of volunteer coordinators are described in Table 23.

Home Health Aides

Home heath aides are central to the provision of hospice/palliative care in the home care setting; they provide most of the patient's physical care and, often, much of the patient's and family's emotional and spiritual support. Patients and families have indicated that home health aides are one of the most valued services provided by hospice/palliative care programs.[107] Because home health aides generally are in the patient's home more frequently than other team members and provide intimate personal care, they are

---

Table 23: Functions of Volunteer Coordinators[90]

Functions Include:

- Administer volunteer programs
- Recruit, screen, train, supervise, and evaluate volunteers
- Maintain records of volunteer references, training, hours, services provided, and evaluations
- Coordinate and facilitate continuing education programs for volunteers
- Coordinate speaker's training sessions for volunteers
- Coordinate volunteer recognition activities
- Educate lay public about hospice concepts and volunteer needs
- Attend IDT meetings
- Work with other team members to assess patient's and family's volunteer needs

likely to be aware of the patient's deepest concerns and can observe family dynamics on a regular basis. See Table 24 for many of the functions and qualification of home health aides.

Specialized Team Members

To meet specific patient needs, specialized healthcare professionals can suggest or provide interventions to improve the patient's and family's quality of life and can educate other team members about the therapeutic benefits of particular interventions. The Medicare Hospice Benefit mandates physical, occupational, and speech therapy services when needed to control symptoms or maintain activities of daily living and basic functional skills.[106] Pharmacists can monitor medication profiles, advise on potential drug interactions, anticipate side effects, and suggest and prepare effective formulations.[80] Music and art therapists can recommend or provide interventions that facilitate life review, enhance relaxation, and provide distraction from distressing symptoms.[80] Specialized team members include:

- Pharmacists
- Art and music therapists

Table 24: Functions and Qualifications of Home Health Aides[106]

Functions Include:

- Observe, document, and report patient status
- Maintain clean, safe environment
- Read and record temperature, pulse, and respirations
- Help patients to self-administer medications
- Perform appropriate, safe patient hygiene and grooming
- Perform basic range of motions and positioning

Qualifications Include:

- Good communication skills
- Good observation skills
- Respect for privacy and property
- Positive attitude

- Occupational and physical therapists
- Respiratory therapists
- Dietitians

Coping with Stress

Hospice/palliative care programs are experiencing challenges similar to those occurring throughout the healthcare system, for example, emphasis on the financial bottom line, downsizing, corporate buyouts, accusations of fraud, refusal to reimburse for nonprocedure-related care (especially psychosocial and spiritual care), pressure to shorten visits and see more patients in less time, and rapid proliferation of competing programs vying for patients, dollars, and community recognition.[108] Rapid changes in the healthcare system contribute to physician stress, as do difficult patients, stressful life events, and professional challenges.

Difficult Patients

Difficult patients and family members present their own set of challenges. When physicians must care for patients they do not like, it is important to acknowledge the following:[109]

- Not all terminally patients are calm, intelligent, and friendly; some are abusive and manipulative.
- Physicians are not always the cause of a patient's or family member's anger. More often anger results from displaced fear, anxiety, and a sense of helplessness in the face of serious illness and approaching death.
- Physicians are likely to experience some degree of dislike, anger, and revulsion when confronted with abusive or manipulative patients or family members who are less than honest and refuse to implement agreed-upon interventions.
- Physicians are likely to avoid patients and family members they do not like, then feel guilty about not establishing a therapeutic relationship.
- Not only is it difficult to establish therapeutic relationships with angry, abusive patients and family members; it is also difficult to establish and maintain even a professional relationship, which is the required minimum.

When faced with patients they do not like, physicians can try the following strategies:[109]

- Make a conscious effort to find a connection with the patient, even if it is just a geographic one.

- Deliberately use communication strategies to draw patients out and learn their stories, which may shed light on their behavior and allow the physician to, if not like a particular patient, at least gain better understanding of the person's behavior.

- Use self-knowledge, self-monitoring, and self-evaluation to better understand personal issues that are contributing to strong emotional reactions to certain patients.

When it becomes clear that, regardless of the physician's best efforts, a satisfying patient–physician relationship is not going to occur, physicians can try the following strategies:[109]

- Establish some emotional distance from the patient.

- Concentrate on acting in a professional manner.

- Take time for self-care activities to reduce stress and maintain some sense of perspective.

- Involve other team members, some of whom might be able to develop more effective relationships with specific patients.

- Refer the patient to another physician if necessary.

Stress Overload

Most physicians view themselves as much more than technicians and purveyors of pills and procedures and are troubled when they cannot establish satisfying relationships with patients and family members. In most cases, a natural sense of empathy underlies a physician's professional interest in patients. The same sense of empathy enhances the physician's ability to listen, offer guidance, relieve fears, and provide emotional support as patients and families search for a renewed sense of hope, purpose, and meaning. However, when too many stressors occur simultaneously, stress overload compromises a physician's judgment and interferes with the ability to interact compassionately with patients, families, and co-workers. Table 25 lists organizational, professional, and personal stressors frequently associated with stress overload. Table 26 describes signs and symptoms of stress overload in physicians.

Table 25: Factors Associated with Stress Overload in Physicians[110]

Personal Variables

■ *Age*. Young age is associated with more stress, fewer coping mechanisms, and more burnout.

■ *Personality*. People with hardy personalities often cope better with work-related stress. They view change as a normal challenge that contributes to further development. Hardy personalities are characterized by the following: commitment, challenge, curiosity about life and meaningfulness, and a sense of being able to influence events.

■ *Motivation for career choice*. Paradoxically, the reasons for choosing palliative medicine can contribute to stress overload. For example, a desire to help others contributes to stress when the physician's help is not wanted or appreciated. In some cases, physicians devote so much energy to their patients that they have none left for themselves or their own family members.[111]

■ *Social supports*. Physicians who use only their own family members for emotional support and debriefing are likely to experience difficulties when family members are unable or unwilling to continue providing sole support, e.g., when family members experience their own crises.

■ *Life events*. Stressful life events, e.g., family illness, bereavement, or relationship problems, create additional stress.

Role Difficulties

■ Role ambiguity, excessive responsibility, and role conflict create stress.

Communication Problems

■ Communication problems with peers, team members, patients, the patient's family members, and the physician's own family members contribute to stress.

■ Difficulty expressing deep pain and grief when interventions fail to relieve a patient's suffering or when favorite patients die can lead to unexpressed, unacknowledged grief that accumulates over time.

Organizational Stresses

■ Inadequate resources and staffing

■ Professional isolation and the loneliness associated with practicing in a developing field of medicine

■ Conflicts with program managers and/or owners

Stress Management Strategies

When caring for terminally ill patients, physicians must learn to acknowledge their own needs and anticipate the inevitable occurrence of psychological and spiritual issues that will cause them personal distress. When events threaten to overwhelm their resources

> ## Table 26: Signs and Symptoms of Stress Overload in Physicians[110,112]
>
> - Tiredness out of proportion to the work that is being done
> - Low morale
> - Overconscientiousness, loss of a sense of proportion, and preoccupation with patients
> - Loss of sense of humor
> - Conflicts with staff and scapegoating
> - Avoidance of patients
> - Difficulties at home
> - Distancing, depersonalization, and intellectualization
> - Anger, irritability, frustration
> - Helplessness, inadequacy, and insecurity
> - Depression, grief, and guilt
> - Errors in judgment

for coping, physicians need to recognize the importance of the following: (1) ministering to body, mind, and spirit, (2) making specific plans for self-care, and (3) acting on these plans. Strategies such as those described in Table 27 can help to reduce stress and enhance personal and professional growth.

With the help of self-care activities and spiritual practices such as nature appreciation, journaling, contemplative prayer, meditation, or yoga, physicians can learn to transcend their own role attachments and co-exist with their very normal feelings of fear, guilt, and grief. Physicians who accept their own periodic bouts of psychological and spiritual distress are better able to empathize with the psychic pain experienced by terminally ill patients as they try to come to terms with loss in new and more meaningful ways.

Dr. Cicely Saunders frequently reminds physicians that dying patients need the support of a caring community *and* the community needs the insights of dying patients. As healthcare professionals witness the attempts of terminally ill patients to develop a renewed sense of meaning, purpose, and hope, they are frequently inspired to examine their own sources of meaning. Then the opportunities for developing the wisdom that comes from working with dying patients can help physicians to learn to (1) cope with the psychological and spiritual pain that occurs in their own lives, (2) provide better care for all of their patients, and (3) develop their own sources of meaning. Few professional opportunities offer such great rewards.

Table 27: Strategies for Managing Stress[110]

Develop a Sense of Competence

- Develop professional skills, set realistic goals, test competence in a number of different situations, share competence with others.
- Attend palliative medicine conferences.
- Locate resources for assistance with difficult cases, e.g., call the AAHPM for help locating other hospice/palliative care physicians with similar interests.

Develop Practice Patterns That Enhance Control and Pleasure

- Focus on areas of personal interest, schedule appointments so that difficult patients are followed by patients who the physician enjoys.

Develop Decision-making Protocols

- Develop formal decision-making protocols, particularly when making difficult treatment-related decisions.
- Involve others in the decision-making process (see *UNIPAC Six: Ethical and Legal Decision Making When Caring for the Terminally Ill*).

Develop Collegial Relationships with Other Professionals

- Develop supportive relationships with physicians and other healthcare professionals to alleviate isolation and provide sources of professional and emotional support.
- Discuss painful psychological and spiritual issues with others, i.e., interested peers, clergy, counselors.

Develop Staffing Policies That Reduce Stress

- Establish policies that allow adequate time away from the work setting.

Develop a Personal Philosophy That Provides a Sense of Meaning[113]

- Develop a personal philosophy that provides a sense of meaning for illness, death, and the physician's own role.

Develop Strategies That Provide a Sense of Rejuvenation

- Participate in activities that provide a sense of psychological, physical, and spiritual rejuvenation, e.g., meditation, prayer, worship, exercise, or enjoying the outdoors.
- Use religious and spiritual practices to strengthen the clinician's own spiritual resources.
- Spend time with family members, not only doing productive things, but also just being together.
- Participate in activities for their intrinsic enjoyment, not for reward or acclamation, e.g., read nonprofessional literature, listen to or play music, garden, walk, watch birds, or write poetry.

(Continued)

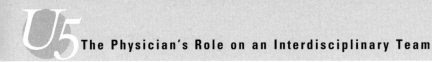

Develop Personal Habits That Increase the Ability to Cope with Stress

- Get adequate sleep and frequent exercise, and develop healthy eating patterns.
- Balance work and home life to avoid exhaustion.
- Use counseling to gain insights and to help to resolve problems.
- Get enough time off call and take vacations whenever possible.

Acknowledge Life's Imperfections

- Acknowledge the likelihood of periodic challenges to the clinician's own psychological and spiritual equilibrium.
- Recognize limitations and the inability to ensure a perfect outcome for every patient and family.
- Recognize that effectively using available knowledge and resources, providing caring presence, and referring to team members and consultants is all that can be done.

If Necessary, Find New Professional Opportunities

- When coping mechanisms fail and external situations cannot be changed, it may be necessary to leave unhealthy work situations and find other, more satisfying, professional opportunities.

Engel argues that the most necessary and the most complex skills of the physician are the ability to elicit an accurate verbal account of the patient's illness experience and then to analyze it properly. He believes that it takes a careful discipline to develop reliable skills in the interviewing process and to understand "the meaning" of the patient's report in psychological, social and cultural as well as anatomical, physiological, or biochemical terms.

—ENGEL, QUOTED IN WILLIAMSON AND NOEL[114]

Stories are medicine. . . . They have such power; they do not require that we do, be, act anything—we need only listen. The remedies for repair or reclamation of any lost psychic drive are contained in stories. Stories engender the excitement, sadness, questions, longings, and understandings that spontaneously bring the archetype back to the surface. . . . Stories set the inner life into motion, and this is particularly important where the inner life is frightened, wedged, or cornered. Story greases the hoists and pulleys, it causes adrenaline to surge, shows us the way out, down, or up, and for our trouble, cuts for us fine wide doors in previously blank walls, openings that lead to the dreamland, that lead to love and learning, that lead us back to our own real lives.

—CLARISSA PINKOLA ESTÉS[115]

Effective training techniques for improving communication include those listed in Table 28; however, skills training alone may not be enough. Beneficial behavior changes are more likely to occur when skills training is coupled with exercises that enhance personal growth and awareness.[116]

As patients and their physicians confront the unfathomable mysteries of life and death, hospice/palliative medicine requires:

- Excellent skills in palliative medicine

- An ability to communicate with honesty and compassion

- An ability to work with other healthcare professionals to alleviate the physical, emotional, spiritual, and social contributors to the suffering often experienced by terminally ill patients and their families

- An abiding interest in patients and their stories[119]

(AAHPM

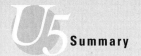

Table 28: Training for Effective Communication

- Read books and attend conferences on effective communication.[117]
- Use interactive CD-ROM discs and other video recordings instead of audio tapes because they illustrate nonverbal communication more effectively[118]
- Attend small-group training sessions on effective communication.
- Video record interactions with simulated patients and receive feedback from experienced facilitators.
- Video record interactions with terminally ill patients and receive feedback from experienced facilitators.

- An ability to let go of the need to always be in control
- A willingness to periodically let go of the role of teacher and become the student

Alleviating a terminally ill patient's physical, emotional, spiritual, and social pain requires excellent communication skills and an interdisciplinary team approach to care. As dying patients struggle to find a renewed sense of meaning, purpose, value, self-worth, and hope for their lives, they want to understand their illness not only cognitively, but also emotionally and spiritually. They want more than facts about their diagnosis, prognosis, and treatment plan—they want guidance, compassionate understanding, and a chance to tell their stories. In the midst of all the talking that goes on in their lives, patients long for understanding and for the deep emotional and spiritual healing that accompanies true communication and the sense of being heard.

Communicating Bad News

Eleanor and James G.

Eleanor G. is a 43-year-old hospice/palliative care patient whose husband, James, owns a profitable building company. During the first 11 years of their marriage, Eleanor and James concentrated on their careers and waited to have children until Eleanor was 35 years of age. Now they have three young children: Mark is 7, Melissa is 5, and Robert is 3. Eleanor sometimes misses the intellectual stimulation of her career as a stockbroker and had planned to return to work when her children were school-aged.

A year ago, Eleanor was diagnosed with cervical cancer, for which she received radiation and chemotherapy, but the cancer spread locally. Several months ago, Eleanor was admitted to a hospice/palliative care program, where she has received medical therapy for pain and emotional support from the home care team. Although Eleanor feels tired much of the time and has enrolled Robert in a part-time day-care center so that she can rest in the mornings, she can still move around the house independently and provide most of the children's care.

Recently, James began to help more and now drives the children to school and day care. In general, the family is coping fairly well.

During the course of her illness, Eleanor has experienced periodic bouts of increased physical pain. Good palliative management has controlled her symptoms, so she does not associate increased discomfort with rapidly approaching death. Despite her professional interest in financial planning, Eleanor has not made a will or planned for her own funeral.

Because Eleanor is still able to participate in the ongoing management of the household, she copes with her emotional distress by avoiding the long-term implications of her illness. She has not made plans for the children's care after her death. Eleanor's physical symptoms are well controlled, so the nurse has been visiting once every 2 weeks; but the chaplain has been visiting weekly due to concerns about Eleanor's apparent unwillingness to consider the implications of her situation. Eleanor seems to enjoy the chaplain's visits, but limits her conversation to the weather, her children's school activities, and her physical symptoms.

One morning the hospice/palliative care program's staff physician, Dr. Davis, receives an urgent call from the nurse, who reports that Eleanor is experiencing substantially increased pain, weakness, and general distress. Despite the nurse's careful description of Eleanor's symptoms, Dr. Davis is uncertain about what is happening and is concerned that Eleanor's condition may have taken a turn for the worse.

Question One

At this point, which responses are the best course of action for the physician? Choose all that apply.

A. Prescribe an increase in Eleanor's baseline dose of slow-release morphine and the dose of immediate-release morphine for breakthrough pain.

B. Ask the nurse to schedule a physician home visit for that afternoon so that Dr. Davis can examine Eleanor alone, without distressing James.

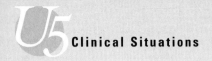

C. Ask the nurse to talk with Eleanor about her changed condition and suggest the urgent need to make funeral plans.

D. Ask the nurse to set up a physician home visit for that afternoon at a time when James can be home; then Dr. Davis will examine Eleanor and visit with both of them.

- Eleanor and James can discuss the news together after Dr. Davis leaves. Due to the distressing nature of the news, neither of them is likely to remember all the information, but they will have a better chance of remembering important points and thinking of questions to ask if they are both present during the interview.

Correct Responses and Analysis

The correct responses are A and D. Response A is correct because Eleanor's pain needs to be addressed immediately and an increase in opioids is likely to help, regardless of additional medications that might also be needed. Response D is correct because Eleanor's changed condition requires reassessment and a careful history and physical, and because a family member or friend should be present. (See the following note.) Response B is incorrect because patients need a family member or friend to provide emotional support when physicians communicate bad news, and because excluding James from the process will isolate him and reinforce Eleanor's tendency to keep her concerns to herself. C is incorrect because it forces the nurse to assume the physician's responsibility for communicating with the patient and because it is premature; the physician has not yet assessed the situation.

NOTE: Because Dr. Davis strongly suspects the need to communicate bad news about Eleanor's changed condition, James needs to be present so that:

- Eleanor will have emotional support when she hears the bad news.

- Eleanor, James, and Dr. Davis can discuss the changed situation and its implications for the family.

The Case Continues

A home visit is scheduled for late that afternoon. During the history phase of the interview, Dr. Davis asks Eleanor to describe how things have been over the past several days. Eleanor says that she has been feeling progressively worse for 2 days and fell while she was trying to get out of bed. Since the fall, she has remained in bed, where she has had more back pain and decreased sensation in her legs.

When Dr. Davis asks Eleanor what she thinks is going on, Eleanor says that at first she thought she had a cold, but then she noticed she couldn't move her legs. As soon as she mentions her legs, Eleanor bursts into tears. Dr. Davis waits quietly until Eleanor's nonverbal communication indicates that she is ready for a tissue. After handing Eleanor the tissue and waiting until Eleanor is ready to talk, Dr. Davis validates Eleanor's feelings by saying the increased weakness and uncertainty must be very difficult to cope with. Again, Dr. Davis gently asks Eleanor what she thinks is going on and waits for her response. When Eleanor says she just doesn't know, Dr. Davis suggests a quick exam, after which they may know more. Eleanor agrees, her eyes full of tears.

The physical exam reveals increased cachexia and anxiety, increased pain and tenderness in the lower lumbar–upper sacral area, and considerably decreased sensation and severe motor weakness from the waist down. Eleanor's symptoms indicate the onset of hemiplegia, probably due to spinal cord involvement. The symptoms suggest that the disease is advanced, pain is going to be difficult to control, and Eleanor is unlikely to be able to walk again or provide much physical care for her children. The physician quickly considers steroids and radiation therapy, but recalls that Eleanor has already been radiated in the affected area. The physician doubts that surgery can reverse such dense hemiplegia in such a sick cancer patient. Surgery would also result in hospitalization, which is Eleanor's greatest fear because it will separate her from her children.

During previous visits with hospice/palliative staff, Eleanor has acknowledged her advanced cervical cancer but, due to her relatively symptom free state, she hasn't seen it as causing a problem in the near future and has avoided discussing the long-term implications of her illness.

Question Two

At this point, which is the best course of action for the physician?

A. Quickly communicate everything Eleanor should know about her condition and its implications because she must make plans for her immediate future.

B. Provide some basic information ("fire a warning shot"), and wait to see how Eleanor responds before talking about the implications of Eleanor's condition.

C. Honor Eleanor's previous denial by avoiding discussions of her condition and its implications.

D. Discuss the news privately with James to protect Eleanor from the bad news about her changed condition.

Correct Response and Analysis

The best response is B. During the history phase of the interview, Dr. Davis asked questions that provided information about how much Eleanor knows and how much she wants to know. Eleanor suspects that her situation is grim and is fearful of hearing bad news. Dr. Davis needs to prepare James and Eleanor for the bad news, then gently share information about Eleanor's changed condition so that they can ask questions about its meaning and begin making decisions about the future, when they are ready to do so. The type and amount of information that Dr. Davis communicates will depend on Eleanor's response; she still may not be ready to consider the implications of her changed condition.

Response A is incorrect because it is important to share information in small steps and assess the patient's reactions. Although Eleanor's situation is serious, she may not be ready to hear the full implications of her condition during this interview. Sharing unwanted information is counterproductive; patients are unable to integrate it, and they are likely to feel as if their needs are being ignored and they are being assaulted with unwanted news by an uncaring physician. C is incorrect because the situation has changed dramatically, and Dr. Davis needs to give Eleanor the opportunity to hear additional information. D is incorrect because excluding Eleanor automatically shuts her out of the decision-making process.

The Case Continues

Dr. Davis decides to provide some basic information and a possible treatment plan and then wait to see how Eleanor and James respond. Although Eleanor and James need information about Eleanor's changed condition, it is unlikely that

Eleanor will want to consider all the ramifications of the current crisis at this time, because she is still in some physical pain, is emotionally distressed, and is likely to continue using denial as a coping technique. There is no need for Dr. Davis to cover everything during this interview: communication is an ongoing process and the family will have other opportunities to talk with the physician. James may want to know more about the meaning of Eleanor's symptoms so that he can plan for the family's immediate future.

After giving Eleanor an additional dose of immediate-release morphine and helping her to find a comfortable position in bed, Dr. Davis sits down and gently suggests that the situation has changed for the worse. Dr. Davis tells Eleanor and James that the new symptoms are a serious complication that is related to the cancer. The physician relates suspicions that the cancer has affected the nerves in Eleanor's legs and briefly describes the options of radiation and surgery. Dr. Davis does not recommend these options, saying that they are unlikely to be very helpful in this situation and will result in Eleanor's separation from her family. Dr. Davis explains that more can be done to control Eleanor's pain and suggests that steroids may temporarily bring back some leg strength. Then Dr. Davis pauses, asks Eleanor if she has any questions, and waits to see how she responds. Eleanor considers the information for a while, then looks at the physician and asks when she will be able to walk again.

Question Three

At this point, what is the physician's best response?

A. You'll never be able to walk again.

B. There's no need to talk about that now. Let's see how things go.

C. You never know, you could be up and around in a few days.

D. We will try the steroids, but I'm concerned that the strength in your legs may not come back completely.

Correct Response and Analysis

The correct response is D, which communicates the physician's concern, provides another warning shot about the seriousness of Eleanor's condition, suggests that Eleanor is unlikely to regain complete use of her legs, and leaves the door open for some degree of hope. While response A may be factually correct, it is unnecessarily harsh and precludes all hope. Response B is evasive and dismissive, and C is misleading because it is overly optimistic.

The Case Continues

Dr. Davis explains that steroids can be used at home and might provide some short-term improvement, but their effects are likely to be temporary and may not be enough to help Eleanor to walk. Dr. Davis's suggestion offers some realistic hope for short-term improvement, but stresses its temporary nature and its limited effects on Eleanor's ability to walk.

Again, Dr. Davis asks if there are questions. Eleanor focuses solely on the steroid treatments. After responding to all Eleanor's questions, Dr. Davis says, "All of this must be overwhelming and hard to think about. I wonder if you have other questions about how all of this is likely to affect you and your family." Eleanor responds by saying that she is tired and doesn't want to talk anymore. Before leaving the room, Dr. Davis sympathizes with Eleanor about everything that is happening to her and closes with, "I want you to know that I am going to stick with you. The hospice/palliative care team will be visiting much more frequently. We will continue to focus on controlling your symptoms, and will order a special mattress to protect your skin and make the bed softer and more comfortable. Even though all of us on the team will be making more regular visits, please don't hesitate to call my office or the program office if you have any questions or just want to talk. I hope we can begin thinking about the future and making some plans. I'll be in the kitchen writing some orders if you think of other questions."

By remaining in the house instead of leaving immediately, physicians provide family members with an opportunity to ask questions that they are reluctant to voice in front of the patient. This is particularly important when patients do not want to discuss the implications of their condition. Dr. Davis orders a special bed, an increased dose of slow-release morphine, dexamethasone, and an antidepressant such as doxepin (Sinequan) to help to relieve nerve-damage pain.

James joins Dr. Davis in the kitchen and asks what Eleanor's condition means in terms of time and her ability to care for their children. Dr. Davis notes the impossibility of making accurate predictions, but provides James with a general framework by saying that Eleanor probably has only a few more weeks to live. When James asks if that means 2 weeks, Dr. Davis responds that it is impossible to know for sure, but Eleanor is likely to live more than a few days and less than a few months.

The physician's response reinforces Eleanor's limited life expectancy without predicting a specific number of days or weeks, which is likely to be wrong. Family members often view specific numbers as certainties and are upset when patients die earlier or live longer than the physician predicted.

Dr. Davis also mentions that Eleanor is likely to experience periods of drowsiness and confusion. It would be wise to arrange for someone to help to care for the children and be with Eleanor as much as possible. When James says Eleanor's mother has offered to help for a few weeks whenever she is needed, Dr. Davis suggests calling her now. Dr. Davis plans to make another home visit in 2 weeks, but asks James to call if Eleanor's condition changes.

James now has some important information that Eleanor does not have, but Dr. Davis did not purposely exclude Eleanor or withhold information. Instead, Dr. Davis provided Eleanor with several opportunities to ask for more information. Eleanor declined them because she is not yet ready to think about the implications of her condition. It would be unkind and counterproductive to force Eleanor to listen to information that she does not want to hear. By giving James an opportunity to ask for more information, Dr. Davis acknowledges that, in some cases, families want more information, or different types of information, than do patients.

Although Eleanor has indicated that she is not ready to discuss the implications of the current crisis, she may be ready to do so in the next several days. Because Eleanor has established a close relationship with the chaplain, Mike, Dr. Davis calls Mike, describes the situation, and asks him to visit with Eleanor as frequently as possible. Patients are more likely to discuss their deepest concerns with the member of the team with whom they feel particularly close.

The next day the nurse calls to report that Eleanor's pain is much improved with the increased slow-release morphine, dexamethasone, and doxepin. During the next 2 weeks, Dr. Davis receives frequent reports from the nurse and the chaplain about Eleanor's condition. During team meetings, Mike reports that he and Eleanor have been reviewing Eleanor's life, discussing what has been most important to her, and talking about the distress she feels because she is unable to physically care for her children. When Mike asked Eleanor if the social worker could visit with the children, she agreed. When he asked her if she had thought about leaving something for the children, such as a letter, or if she had thought about plans for the children's schooling, Eleanor became very quiet and eventually said she probably needed to start thinking about things like that. Then she quickly shifted the discussion to the weather, baseball, and the family's plans to have an indoor picnic.

The social worker reports that she has visited with the children several times to talk with them about their mother's illness and to address their concerns and fears. She is concerned because neither Eleanor nor James will talk with the children about Eleanor's coming death. She recommends that the team continue to provide emotional support for Eleanor, James, and the children and suggests that Eleanor needs to talk with her children about her illness and about the future.

As promised, the physician visits in 2 weeks. Eleanor is glad to see Dr. Davis and seems to be in a different emotional and spiritual place than she was during the previous visit. Her increased disability and ongoing visits with the chaplain are gradually helping her to accept her illness in ways that the physician could not have done in the previous visit. Dr. Davis sits down and asks Eleanor about her condition. Eleanor indicates her pain is better, rates the pain as 4 on a 10-point scale, says she is able to sleep through the night, and reports that she is rarely hungry, wanting only a few bites of soft food a couple of times a day. Eleanor's condition is clearly deteriorating. She is now completely bedbound and is periodically disoriented and confused.

When Dr. Davis asks Eleanor to describe how she is feeling otherwise, Eleanor looks into the physician's eyes and says, "I'm not going to be here much longer, am I?"

Question Four

At this point, which of the following is the best response?

A. "Eleanor, I think you may be right."

B. "Of course you aren't, that's what we've been trying to tell you all along!"

C. "Can you tell me more about what you mean?"

D. "Who knows? We're all terminal, and none of us knows when we're going to die."

Correct Response and Analysis

The best response is probably C. It is likely that Eleanor is asking for information about her prognosis, but jumping to conclusions is dangerous. Response A could be an appropriate response to a direct question, such as "Am I dying?" Response B is sarcastic and judgmental. Response D is superficial and patronizing.

The Case Continues

In response to Dr. Davis's request for more information, Eleanor says that she knows she is dying and wants to know how much longer she will live.

At this point, Eleanor deserves a clear response to the deeply distressing question that she has been avoiding for months. Answering Eleanor as clearly as possible acknowledges the courage it took for her to ask the question. By gently agreeing with Eleanor's conclusion that she is dying, Dr. Davis confirms Eleanor's suspicions, supports Eleanor's feelings of worth by indicating that Eleanor has come to a correct conclusion, and indicates that it is okay for Eleanor to talk about her coming death.

After gently agreeing with Eleanor, Dr. Davis asks Eleanor what else is on her mind. Eleanor responds by saying that James and the children are talking about a family cruise on the Caribbean as soon as school is out, in about a month. She is concerned because the tickets are nonrefundable and wonders if it might be better to see how she is feeling before buying the tickets. Dr. Davis gently confirms that Eleanor is right; delaying the purchase is probably wise because she may not feel like going on a long trip.

Eleanor begins to cry quietly, and the physician waits for Eleanor's emotions to subside. When Eleanor recovers, Dr. Davis acknowledges that Eleanor is going through a difficult time that would be upsetting for anyone. The physician asks Eleanor what else is on her mind and waits for Eleanor's response. After a few minutes, Eleanor asks what it will be like to die.

Question Five

Which of the following is the best response?

A. Most people become more and more drowsy and eventually die in their sleep.

B. Let's face that when it arrives.

C. Can you tell me something about your main worries?

D. Don't worry about the future.

Correct Response and Analysis

The best response is C. Patients have a wide range of worries, and there is no way of knowing which are particularly bothersome for a specific patient

without asking. When physicians respond with open questions, patients are encouraged to identify and acknowledge their main concerns. Then physicians can offer therapeutic support, reassurance that such concerns are normal, and factual information as needed. Response A is factual, but may not address this patient's main concerns; B is evasive and dismissive. D is neither empathetic nor as helpful as C in this particular situation.

The Case Concludes

Eleanor responds that she is most fearful of pain. Dr. Davis reassures her that the medications will be increased as needed and that other techniques will be used if the tablets stop working well enough. Then Dr. Davis tells Eleanor that most patients become more and more drowsy and eventually die in their sleep. Dr. Davis asks Eleanor if there are things she would like to finish up in the next several days or week. When Eleanor says she is not sure, Dr. Davis gently suggests that she might want to hug her family a lot, tell them how much she loves them, talk with her children about their future, and tell them who will be taking care of them. Dr. Davis also mentions that the social worker and chaplain can help Eleanor with ideas about how to talk with her children. Eleanor nods, thinks for a while, then comments on the lovely spring weather.

Physicians need to recognize and honor a patient's desire to end a discussion, which is usually communicated with abrupt changes in conversation or with more direct comments such as, "Thank you for coming by to see me. . . . Don't forget your umbrella on your way out. . . . My husband will help you find the door."

Because the thought of leaving young children is almost unbearable for parents, parents who are terminally ill often have a particularly difficult time accepting the fact that their life expectancy is limited. Except in rare cases, caregivers should honor the pace at which patients want to discuss their situation. It is rarely necessary or helpful to force patients to confront subjects that they are not yet ready to discuss—sometimes families do need to purchase nonrefundable tickets. However, when single parents refuse to plan for their children's future, more insistence is appropriate, at least until they identify who will be caring for their children after their death.

Two weeks later, Eleanor deteriorates rapidly and is switched to subcutaneous administration of an infusion of hydromorphone (Dilaudid) and haloperidol (Haldol) and to rectal administration of doxepin (Sinequan) capsules to control her increasing neuropathic pain and delirium. (See UNIPACs Three and Four.) Eleanor dies peacefully a week later with her family and the chaplain by her side.

A Family-centered Approach to Care

Aaron Goldman and Family

The phone call is from the hospice/palliative care program's patient care coordinator, who is in a patient's home for an admission visit. The family is distraught. The patient, Aaron, is an 82-year-old German Jew. Aaron had been hospitalized so that doctors could search for the cause of his gradual decline over the past 2 months. When given a diagnosis of end-stage renal disease, the entire family was shocked, first by the diagnosis of end-stage renal disease, then by Aaron's dramatic personality change. He has withdrawn and no longer responds to the family. Will you come and talk with them?

The patient's home is 15 miles out in the country but, fortunately, it's not far off the highway on this rainy evening. Aaron's son-in-law, Marvin, greets you at the back door and ushers you to the kitchen table, where introductions are quickly exchanged. You barely have time to sip the coffee they offer, when Isobel, who is Aaron's eldest daughter, begins telling her father's story. Also present are her sister, Miriam, and her daughter, Rebecca, who, with Marvin, offer occasional supportive comments. Aaron is in the bedroom, yet unseen.

"I need to know, did the hospital kill my father or did I? Last week, he was walking and talking normally, at least for him. We took him to the hospital to find out why his legs hurt so badly. They tell us his kidneys are shot, but no one ever mentioned his kidneys before. The kidney specialist says he is not a candidate for dialysis. The surgeon says the only way to help the pain in his legs is to amputate them. Dad says he wants to

come home. So we bring him home, and he goes to bed, refuses to eat, and will hardly say a word to us. The social worker at the hospital tells us we need hospice. We didn't even know he was dying. What is going on?"

Question One

At this point, which of the following responses are likely to be effective? Choose all that apply.

A. This is certainly a complex situation. Do you think Mr. Goldman would like to be part of this discussion?

B. This whole situation must be overwhelming for you; no wonder you feel frustrated and want to know what's going on. We have a lot to talk about. Can each of you briefly describe your main concern?

C. Your father seems to have poor circulation to his legs and to his kidneys from hardening of the arteries, or arteriosclerosis, which develops slowly over many years. We don't know why he has gotten so sick so fast.

D. Lots of difficulties exist within the medical care triage system. According to the chart, the problem stems from the fact that Mr. Goldman was first seen in the ER, then referred to a surgeon who did an on-the-spot vascular workup. Then you were referred to the in-house physician, who went off call and handed care over to a partner. Then you saw a nephrologist and were discharged to a hospice program that you didn't know anything about. Unfortunately,

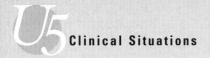

today's medical system is so fragmented, patients and family members are frequently left in the dark about what is going on.

Correct Responses and Analysis

The most effective responses are likely to be A, B, or C because they acknowledge the family's appropriate feelings of frustration and anxiety and its need to make sense of distressing events. Response A encourages the family to consider Mr. Goldman's wishes. Response B encourages family members to identify their own concerns, which will help the physician to decide which issues to address first. Discussing specific concerns will help to alleviate the family's sense of being completely overwhelmed by events. Response C provides needed information about Mr. Goldman's diagnosis and acknowledges the uncertainties related to his prognosis. Response D may be factually correct, but it is unlikely to meet the family's current needs. When patients and families are anxious and worried, they are rarely interested in philosophical discussions about the healthcare system.

The Case Continues

You ask if it would be appropriate to continue the story in Aaron's presence. The family is not sure. With their permission, you go to the bedroom, introduce yourself, and quickly assess that Aaron Goldman is awake and oriented, though noncommittal about being a part of the discussion. Aware of your own personal time constraints, you recognize the risk of forcing the situation, but rationalize to yourself that the current "window of lucidity" is temporary and may not remain open. The family gathers in the bedroom and sits comfortably around the bed.

Mr. Goldman is propped up and given a drink of water. Isobel continues the story. Her father came to this country with six siblings in the late 1920s, settled in the Northeast, found work in a local factory, and met his wife in the local synagogue. Although the marriage was somewhat arranged, the couple's bonds of love and affection were strong from the beginning. The extended family was close and industrious, and their efforts soon evolved into a successful cleaning business. Isobel's father was headstrong and fiercely independent—"an arrogant old German," Isobel says affectionately. His recent willingness to let her do things for him was strong evidence of just how much he was suffering.

Mr. Goldman looks at you without expression or comment, then closes his eyes.

Isobel continues. Twenty years ago, following bypass surgery, Mr. Goldman's toe was partially amputated and he was cautioned that he would eventually lose his leg if he did not quit smoking. He quit.

In recent years, Aaron's wife became increasingly debilitated by osteoporosis and was ultimately wheelchair bound. Aaron, then in retirement, became her caregiver, doing all the shopping, cooking, and cleaning, as well as attending to her personal needs. About 2 years ago, the children noted that after Aaron stood up for awhile his feet turned very dark. Only occasionally would he reveal the intensity of his pain to them, but never to his wife. At times they resented her demanding invalidism, while admiring his tireless devotion.

Aaron looks at Isobel, then at you, and asks, "Are you a doctor? Do you have anything in that black bag to put an end to an old man's misery?" The children respond with a chorus of protests. "Dad! Don't talk like that. He doesn't mean it. He's deeply religious. He would never take his own life. See, this is what we mean. Something terrible must have happened to him in the hospital. He would never have said such things otherwise. Come on, Dad, let us get you something to eat. If you don't, the doctor will have to put a feeding tube down you. Come on, Dad."

Question Two

At this point, which of the following are likely to be effective responses? Choose all that apply.

A. Mr. Goldman, can you tell me more about the pain in your feet?

B. I don't believe more food is likely to relieve Mr. Goldman's distress since his kidneys cannot process it well.

C. Mr. Goldman must be transferred immediately to an inpatient psychiatric facility so that around-the-clock suicide prevention measures can be instituted.

D. I hear Mr. Goldman saying that his misery is very severe. We might want to consider a temporary transfer to a hospice inpatient unit for symptom control or a continuous infusion of medications at home to help to relieve his pain and anxiety.

Correct Responses and Analysis

The correct responses are A, B, and D because they redirect the family's attention from premature fears about suicide to specific issues that are affecting Mr. Goldman's quality of life. Response A is likely to elicit information that will result in better pain control. Response B provides information about Mr. Goldman's condition and its likely effects on the efficacy of treatment with artificial nutrition. Response D is correct because either or both of these suggestions may alleviate the misery that is making Mr. Goldman feel desperate enough to mention suicide.

Response C is incorrect because there is no evidence that Mr. Goldman is seriously considering suicide. Better symptom control, coupled with increased emotional and spiritual support, is likely to help Mr. Goldman to develop a renewed sense of meaning and purpose as his life draws to a close. In any case, transferring him to an inpatient psychiatric facility will increase his isolation from his family and may interfere with adequate pain control measures.

The Case Continues

You ask Aaron about his foot pain. (Sometimes patients are puzzled, even suspicious, about interest in their life story. Starting with more traditional health-related questions may be helpful.) When he says his foot is OK, you confirm that the fentanyl patches are firmly adhered.

Then, with an encouraging nod, Isobel continues. "Two months ago, our mother died. One day Dad was up, driving, shopping, cooking. The next, he was practically helpless. We decided to bring him home to live with us. But things have gotten steadily worse. His leg pain got worse. He cried a lot. The doctors at the VA hospital said he was depressed, but depression medicine didn't help. Finally, he said he couldn't stand the pain anymore, and he agreed to go to the local hospital for evaluation."

A tear trickles down Mr. Goldman's cheek. "That was a waste of time. They ran all these tests on me, but nobody bothered to tell me what was going on." Isobel and Miriam look surprised. "All I know is, I don't want to go on living like this. You wouldn't either, Doc. I don't care what the rabbi says, I'm old, I'm in pain all the time, and I'm a burden to my kids. I can't do anything for myself, food tastes bad, and I don't believe there is anything better for me." Mr. Goldman's voice is flat. His eyes flicker briefly, then become lifeless again

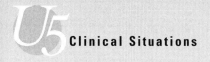

and close in retreat. Isobel and Miriam look at you expectantly.

Question Three

At this point, which of the following are likely to be helpful responses? Choose all that apply.

A. Start a barbiturate infusion to induce unconsciousness at least for a few days.

B. Switch to another opioid without active metabolites, e.g., oxycodone or hydromorphone, and consider a different antidepressant in low doses.

C. Facilitate the telling and recording of Mr. Goldman's life story.

D. Give Mr. Goldman and his family permission to grieve their losses.

Correct Responses and Analysis

Responses B, C, and D are correct; however, to be effective they require involvement of the entire interdisciplinary team as soon as possible. Response B will help to control Mr. Goldman's physical pain (see UNPAC Three), but careful monitoring and instruction by the program's home care nurse is essential during the dose escalation. Responses C and D are likely to alleviate Mr. Goldman's spiritual and emotional pain. Trained volunteers have proved adept at encouraging patients to tell their life stories and recording them, a technique that often leads to a renewed sense of purpose and meaning.[119] Skilled interventions by the program's social worker and chaplain and by Mr. Goldman's rabbi will give Mr. Goldman permission to grieve the loss of his beloved wife, his independence, and his purpose for living. Interventions will also allow Isobel and Miriam to grieve the loss of their mother and the impending loss of their father. The social worker, chaplain, and rabbi can also help Mr. Goldman to continue the developmental tasks of the dying while, at the same time, helping his children to realize that Mr. Goldman has only a short time to live, regardless of which interventions are started.

Response A is incorrect because it is premature. A barbiturate infusion to induce therapeutic sedation is an invaluable tool for relieving intense suffering when all other interventions have failed; however, in this situation, other effective remedies have not yet been tried. (See UNIPACs Two and Four.)

The Case Concludes

During the remainder of the visit, you encourage Mr. Goldman and his family to discuss various options. Mr. Goldman agrees to try additional medications to relieve his pain. Somewhat reluctantly, the family agrees to meet with the program's social worker and chaplain to explore other interventions. You write appropriate orders and give them to the nurse, who will coordinate Mr. Goldman's care.

As soon as practical, you return home, go for a brisk walk, and order nutritious take-out food instead of trying to cook for the family. You ask other family members for help with chores, tell your story, and go to bed as early as possible so that you will have the physical and emotional strength to continue engaging with patients and families on the deepest possible level.

NOTE: An important concept to consider is the impact of the physician's sense of limited time on the outcome of the patient's story. This clinical situation was adapted from a contribution by Charles G. Sasser, MD.

Resolving Team Conflict

Nancy Griffin, MD, Paul Smith, RN, Fred Jones, MD, and Mrs. Fritz

Nancy Griffin, MD, and Paul Smith, RN, are members of an interdisciplinary team at the same hospice/palliative care program. Dr. Griffin is the program's part-time medical director and serves as the attending physician for some of the patients. Paul is a nurse who cares for hospice/palliative care patients in three different nursing homes, all of which contract with the program for end-of-life care services. Dr. Jones is the medical director at the three contracting nursing homes and is the attending physician for Mrs. Fritz, who resides in one of the nursing facilities. Mrs. Fritz is also one of Paul's patients. In the past, Dr. Jones has indicated that he is not particularly interested in palliative care and has voiced concerns about using opioids to control pain.

Mrs. Fritz has been a hospice/palliative care patient for 5 months. She has advanced dementia and congestive heart failure, is bed bound, requires complete assistance with all activities of daily living, and rarely speaks. She has not expressed discomfort from physical pain but occasionally experiences agitation and anxiety, which Dr. Jones treats as needed with lorazepam (Ativan). Over the past 2 days, Paul has become concerned about Mrs. Fritz's increasing restlessness and apparent distress.

When Paul visits on the third day, he finds that Mrs. Fritz is quite agitated and anxious: she is calling out and picking at the air. The nursing home staff is worried that Mrs. Fritz will fall if she climbs over the sides of the bed. Paul listens to Mrs. Fritz's chest and notes increased pulmonary congestion. Paul calls Dr. Jones to report Mrs. Fritz's changed condition. Dr. Jones responds that he just visited Mrs. Fritz a week ago, tells Paul to give the lorazepam as ordered, and abruptly hangs up the phone. Paul watches the nursing home staff try to give Mrs. Fritz the lorazepam pill, but Mrs. Fritz is so agitated and restless she spits it out. Paul calls Dr. Jones's office several more times, but the physician does not come to the phone.

At a hastily convened team meeting, Paul describes his dismay about Mrs. Fritz's condition and expresses his own feelings of irritation and helplessness because Dr. Jones has not returned his calls. Paul knows that other hospice/palliative care patients usually experience relief from regular doses of morphine, so he asks Dr. Griffin to prescribe morphine for Mrs. Fritz, who is clearly in distress.

Question One

What is the best course of action for Dr. Griffin?

A. Remind Paul that Dr. Jones is Mrs. Fritz's attending physician and suggest that he continue his attempts to call Dr. Jones.

B. Remind Paul that it is important not to upset Dr. Jones, because the program does not want to lose its contracts with the nursing homes; suggest that he do the best he can in the situation.

C. Tell Paul that his own distress will not help the situation and remind him that profes-

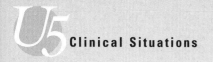
sional etiquette requires that she discuss the situation with Dr. Jones before taking any action.

D. Acknowledge Paul's concern and the urgent need to relieve Mrs. Fritz's distress, remind Paul that professional etiquette requires her to discuss the situation with Dr. Jones before taking any action, and arrange to call Dr. Jones right after the meeting.

Correct Response and Analysis

The correct response is D. Members of effective teams provide emotional support and validation for one another. Paul's distress about Mrs. Fritz's deteriorating condition is appropriate; anyone would feel some degree of helplessness in a similar situation. Dr. Griffin's concern about professional etiquette is also appropriate. Her promise to call Dr. Jones right after the meeting indicates that she is committed to helping Mrs. Fritz and plans to become involved.

The Case Continues

Dr. Griffin calls Dr. Jones, relates Paul's concern, and describes Mrs. Fritz's symptoms. Dr. Jones responds by saying that he has known Mrs. Fritz for a long time, she has these spells occasionally, and if Paul would just follow orders, Mrs. Fritz would eventually calm down. Dr. Griffin asks for permission to do a consultative visit. Dr. Jones pauses, but reluctantly gives permission. Paul is frustrated by this new delay because he wants immediate relief for Mrs. Fritz, but Dr. Griffin says she needs to honor Dr. Jones role as the attending physician and needs to complete a history and physical to determine the best course of action.

That afternoon, when Dr. Griffin arrives at the nursing home, Mrs. Fritz is somewhat less dis-

tressed than she was during Paul's visit. The nursing home staff tells Dr. Griffin that they are concerned about Mrs. Fritz's condition because she has been breathing more heavily, is increasingly confused, and is eating very little. They have contacted Mrs. Fritz's daughter, who plans to arrive in town the next day.

The medical record indicates that Mrs. Fritz's heart failure has been quite severe in the past, requiring intensive treatment on multiple occasions. She has been taking furosemide (Lasix) and digoxin and is on a low-salt diet. Due to her agitation and unwillingness to swallow pills, Mrs. Fritz has taken no medications for the past 2 days. While visiting with Mrs. Fritz, Dr. Griffin notices that she breathes about 35 times per minute and looks distressed. Mrs. Fritz tries to sit up frequently and talks to people who are not there. Dr. Griffin attempts to talk with Mrs. Fritz about her symptoms, but is unsuccessful because Mrs. Fritz is unable to concentrate and ignores the physician's questions.

On physical exam, Dr. Griffin finds an elderly cachectic female with a blood pressure of 105/70, a pulse of 110, and a respiratory rate of 35. The chest exam reveals coarse rales and rhonchi throughout both lower lung fields. Mrs. Fritz has a regular cardiac rhythm with no murmurs, her abdomen is soft but not tender, her extremities show severe muscle wasting, and she has a Stage II decubitus on her sacrum and Stage I decubitus on her heels. Like Paul, Dr. Griffin determines that Mrs. Fritz's heart failure is worsening and may be contributing to her agitated delirium. The patient is clearly in distress from the clouded sensorium, dyspnea, and decubiti.

Dr. Griffin calls Dr. Jones's office. The nurse says she will tell Dr. Jones about the call, but Dr. Griffin receives no response. Dr. Griffin calls again, writes a full consultative note, and faxes it to Dr.

Jones's office. The note includes the following suggestions:

- Injectable furosemide (Lasix) 40 mg SC to help to relieve Mrs. Fritz's pulmonary edema. (Intramuscular injections are discouraged in end-of-life care situations due to the additional pain that they cause. Dr. Griffin believes a few SC injections might relieve Mrs. Fritz's dyspnea and calm the delirium enough to enable her to resume oral medications.)

- Haloperidol (Haldol) 1 to 2 mg PO or SC every 4 hours as needed for agitation

The next morning, Mrs. Fritz's daughter arrives at the nursing home and is very upset to find her mother so distressed and agitated. The daughter calls Paul, angrily demanding to know who is caring for her mother. As soon as the daughter hangs up, Paul calls Dr. Griffin, describes the daughter's distress, and asks Dr. Griffin why nothing has been done.

Question Two

Which of the following is Dr. Griffin's best response?

A. "Look, I'm doing the best I can. You need to learn to be more patient."

B. "I know you are frustrated and so am I. Dr. Jones hasn't returned my call. I will page him as soon as we hang up."

C. "I am the doctor here, and I'll handle it my way."

D. "You call the daughter back, tell her to call Dr. Jones and to complain about her mother's care. If she needs to, the daughter can threaten to sue the doctor and the home."

Correct Response and Analysis

The correct response is B. Dr. Griffin acknowledges Paul's feelings of frustration as well as her own, explains what the situation is, and describes the next step that she will take. Responses A, C, and D are incorrect because they are hostile and will only escalate the growing conflict between the two physicians, between Dr. Griffin and Paul, and between Mrs. Fritz's daughter and staff at the nursing home and the hospice/palliative care program. Response D is a last resort because it shifts responsibility for Mrs. Fritz's care from the hospice/palliative care program to the daughter, and it places the daughter in the position of the "troublemaker" who must confront Dr. Jones.

The Case Continues

Dr. Griffin is very uncomfortable. She is now struggling with her own feelings of irritation based on her sense of helplessness: she wants to intervene because she knows Mrs. Fritz is miserable, she believes that Mrs. Fritz's symptoms can be alleviated, and she wants to honor Dr. Jones's position as the attending physician. She also feels pressured by Paul and Mrs. Fritz's daughter, who are becoming increasingly distressed. In addition, Dr. Jones is not returning her calls. In this situation, it is appropriate for the daughter to be upset about her mother's condition and for Dr. Griffin to be uncomfortable and stressed and for Paul to be feeling the same way.

Dr. Griffin calls Dr. Jones's office again and asks that Dr. Jones be paged. When there is no response, Dr. Griffin calls the director of nurses at the nursing home, who has worked with Dr. Jones on a regular basis. She discusses the situation with him, acknowledges Dr. Jones's long-time relationship with Mrs. Fritz, and describes her own desire to continue working with Dr. Jones in the nursing home. Dr. Griffin also expresses her concerns about Mrs. Fritz's well-being and describes the daughter's distress. The director of nursing reports that the staff are quite concerned about Mrs. Fritz and already know that the daughter is angry. He says he will call Dr. Jones and try to persuade him to allow a limited trial of the recommended interventions.

Dr. Griffin then calls Mrs. Fritz's daughter and acknowledges her concern about Mrs. Fritz. She briefly describes what she found during the examination and expresses her belief that Mrs. Fritz can be made more comfortable with medications that will relieve the shortness of breath and agitation. The daughter responds that she is very worried about her mother and just wants to know what is going on.

Question Three

What is the best next step for Dr. Griffin?

A. Tell the daughter that her mother is dying.

B. Ask the daughter to be patient until her mother gets help.

C. Suggest that Dr. Jones is the one who is causing all the problems.

D. Ask the daughter to describe her main concerns about her mother's condition.

Correct Response and Analysis

The correct response is D. Before proceeding with the conversation, Dr. Griffin needs to assess the daughter's main concerns and find out what the daughter wants to do. The other responses are incorrect: A is premature, B is unlikely to calm the daughter, who has every reason to be impatient, and C undermines another team member, Dr. Jones, the attending physician.

The Case Continues

Mrs. Fritz's daughter responds, "I don't want my mother to suffer! I just want her to be comfortable. I know she's old and has been sick for a long time, but I don't want her to be put on machines and poked with needles and kept alive in this terrible condition. I don't want to do anything that will kill her, but I don't want her to suffer."

Dr. Griffin acknowledges the daughter's concerns and says that everyone wants Mrs. Fritz to be as comfortable as possible, including all the staff at the hospice/palliative care program and the nursing home. Dr. Griffin then agrees with the daughter's assessment; Mrs. Fritz has been very sick for several months and has taken a turn for the worse. She says that Mrs. Fritz may be approaching the end of her life and reiterates everyone's desire to make her comfortable, especially now. Dr. Griffin reassures the daughter that the new medications will not kill her mother; they are recognized treatments for relieving shortness of breath and dementia. The daughter is saddened that her mother's life expectancy may be limited, but at the moment all she wants is relief for her mother's distress. She demands to know when the new treatments will begin. Dr. Griffin says they will begin as soon as Dr. Jones initiates them. Dr. Griffin says she will call the daughter back as soon as she knows something. The daughter thanks Dr. Griffin for calling.

In 10 minutes, the director of nursing calls Dr. Griffin to report that Dr. Jones wants Dr. Griffin to assume care for Mrs. Fritz. The director of nursing told Dr. Jones that the problem was escalating— several people were upset, including the daughter. He told Dr. Jones that he either needed to visit right away and calm the daughter while doing something to relieve Mrs. Fritz's increasing distress or turn Mrs. Fritz over to Dr. Griffin and let her deal with the family. Because Dr. Jones was already scheduled to see 10 other patients on the other side of town, he agreed.

NOTE: When attending physicians feel pressured to provide a recommended therapy with which they are uncomfortable, such as using opioids to treat dyspnea, they often turn the patient's care over to the hospice/palliative care physician. In this case, Dr. Jones may have had qualms about using hydrocodone to treat dyspnea or using injectable furosemide (Lasix). He may have perceived the situation as being less problematic than did Paul and Dr. Griffin, or he may have believed that Mrs. Fritz's symptoms could not be relieved with any treatment.

Dr. Griffin immediately gives verbal orders to initiate the new treatments and calls Paul to let him know what has happened and asks him to visit the nursing facility to make sure that Mrs. Fritz's symptoms improve. She also calls Mrs. Fritz's daughter, tells her that Paul is going to the facility, and promises to stop by later that afternoon.

With the new treatment, Mrs. Fritz's sense of respiratory distress is partially relieved and she becomes calmer. The hydrocodone is increased to 8 mg q 4 hours, but Mrs. Fritz is unable to swallow even this small amount of liquid. A 25 mcg per hour fentanyl patch (Duragesic) is applied, and she receives subcutaneous injections of haloperidol (Haldol) 2 mg three times a day. Mrs. Fritz's restlessness and dyspnea subside, she becomes quite drowsy, and her blood pressure decreases, so the furosemide (Lasix) is stopped.

Mrs. Fritz's delirium is now controlled enough that she is able to squeeze her daughter's hand. When the daughter sees that her mother is comfortable, she too becomes calmer. Later, Paul and Dr. Griffin visit with the daughter and explain what is likely to happen over the next couple of days. The daughter thanks them for their help. Mrs. Fritz

dies 2 days later without acute distress, and her daughter expresses her gratitude to Paul and the nursing home staff.

Dr. Griffin follows up with a telephone call and a letter to Dr. Jones stating that Mrs. Fritz died comfortably and the daughter was grateful to the staff of the hospice/palliative care program and the nursing facility for working together to help her mother. Dr. Griffin helps preserve Dr. Jones's sense of integrity by including a consultative note in which she thanks Dr. Jones for the opportunity to be involved in Mrs. Fritz's care. She also includes a copy of the American Academy of Hospice and Palliative Medicine's *Pocket Guide to Hospice/Palliative Medicine*.

When the case is reviewed at the next team conference, Paul reports that he is still distressed over Mrs. Fritz's care and complains that too much time elapsed before Mrs. Fritz's symptoms were controlled. Dr. Griffin feels attacked and accused.

Question Four

Which of the following is the physician's most appropriate response?

A. As soon as Paul stops talking, immediately move on to the next patient, in hopes that ignoring the conflict will make it go away.

B. Tell Paul to relax; the patient's condition eventually improved and now she is dead.

C. Remind Paul that from the time she got involved it was one and a half days until Mrs. Fritz got some relief.

D. Acknowledge her own distress about the case and suggest that the team take a minute to review it in hopes of finding solutions for the future.

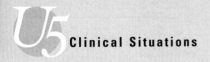

Correct Response and Analysis

Response D is correct. By acknowledging her own distress, Dr. Griffin validates Paul's feelings and aligns herself with Paul. Asking the team to review the situation is more likely to validate Paul's belief that the issue is important and result in healing. By asking the team to concentrate on solutions for the future, Dr. Griffin shifts the focus of the discussion to mutual goals, instead of on who was right or wrong. The other responses are incorrect: A will not resolve the conflict, B is dismissive and hostile, and C doesn't address the real source of Paul's distress.

The Case Concludes

As the team reviews the situation, Paul says that he feels terrible because (1) Mrs. Fritz's symptoms weren't alleviated earlier and he knew what the problem was, (2) he felt helpless because he was ignored first by Dr. Jones, then by Dr. Griffin, and (3) he was very distressed because the daughter and the nursing home staff were questioning his competence and his commitment to his patients.

Dr. Griffin acknowledges Paul's concern for Mrs. Fritz and says that she too had been very concerned about Mrs. Fritz's obvious distress and had done the best she could to relieve the symptoms as quickly as possible. She acknowledges her own temporary feeling of helplessness when Dr. Jones seemed reluctant to consider the new treatments and explains her concern about superseding Dr. Jones's orders: alienating Dr. Jones might compromise the program's access to other terminally ill patients needing help with symptom control.

Dr. Griffin also says she is sorry that all of them had to go through such a difficult time. She suggests that Dr. Jones might have been concerned about using opioids to treat dyspnea because their use is not widely publicized outside palliative care circles. Then Dr. Griffin asks Paul and the rest of the team if they can think of ways to provide more physician education about palliative symptom management. Paul, Dr. Griffin, and the rest of the team identify several possibilities:

- Presentations during Grand Rounds at the local hospital

- A newsletter about symptom control mailed to all community physicians

- An invitational lunch for physicians that includes a lecture on the management of difficult symptoms

- Providing each referring physician with copies of educational materials available from the American Academy of Hospice and Palliative Medicine, such as the *Pocket Guide to Hospice/Palliative Medicine*, and the UNIPAC series, particularly the modules addressing pain and symptom control.

When the discussion ends, Paul thanks Dr. Griffin for her concern and support. Paul and Dr. Griffin acknowledge that stress had affected their ability to respond rationally in a difficult situation.

To relieve her own stress, Dr. Griffin leaves the office a little early, goes for a long jog, and tells her story to her husband that evening. They plan time for Dr. Griffin to get a massage during the coming weekend. She adds an entry to her journal. Then she writes herself a note to ask the hospice/palliative program's director of nursing to thank the nursing home's director of nursing for his help and to offer an inservice on subcutaneous infusions. She uses progressive muscle relaxation exercises to help herself to get to sleep.

Managing Stress

Dr. Claiborne

Jay Claiborne, MD, is a 40-year-old family practice physician who has served as the part-time medical director of a community hospice/palliative care program for 2 years. Although Jay's duties are primarily administrative, he makes consultative home visits when requested for symptom management. Jay chooses to work with dying patients because he enjoys the intimate patient–physician relationships that sometimes develop during the last phases of a patient's life. Jay's work as medical director has also been satisfying for him because the program has grown rapidly and has provided good symptom control and emotional support for patients and family members. Jay also enjoys working as a member of an interdisciplinary team and believes that he is particularly skilled at providing end-of-life care.

At the office, Jay and his two partners are working hard to enlarge their practice. For the past two years, Jay has been able to manage his clinical work and still give two half-days a week to the hospice/palliative care program for minimal compensation. Recently, a managed-care corporation offered the practice several contracts. Jay, his partners, and the corporation have very different ideas about specific contract issues. The differences of opinion are causing some stress within the practice.

Jay and his wife, Katherine, have one child and are expecting a second in 5 months. Their first child was recently diagnosed with learning disabilities requiring expensive intervention. Katherine's pregnancy has been difficult, with lots of nausea and vomiting. Katherine is very concerned about their first child, but does not always feel well enough to interact with him as much as she thinks she should. She is also very concerned about the effects of increased family stress on her career as a college professor.

During the past year and a half, the hospice/palliative care program's daily census gradually expanded to about 90 patients, but in the past 2 months it has suddenly dropped to about 60 patients. A national corporation recently opened a competing program and is conducting a sophisticated marketing campaign to recruit patients. The community program has responded to the financial crisis by terminating patient care staff and hiring an additional marketing person. Jay particularly misses one of the home care nurses and a social worker, both of whom were very supportive of his constant efforts to improve care. Jay now believes the program's quality of care is suffering. He suspects that the program is receiving complaints from physicians, patients, and family members about reductions in home visits and decreases in adequate symptom control. Jay's growing concern about the program is affecting his relationship with the program's administrator.

During a Monday afternoon team meeting, one of the three remaining home care nurses complains that so many patients called over the weekend that she was unable to visit all of them in a timely manner. The nurse is feeling overworked because her patient load has increased to 22 patients and because she had to cover the weekend when one of the on-call nurses was suddenly "no longer with us." She reports that one of Jay's patients called several times because his symptoms were out of control, but she was unable to get to the patient's home until late Sunday afternoon.

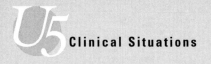

She called Jay's partner, who was covering for Jay over the weekend, but he didn't seem to know what to do.

When Jay hears that a favorite patient from his own practice was suffering from uncontrolled symptoms, he experiences a surge of overwhelming anger and guilt. He makes a derogatory comment about the program's deteriorating quality of care and abruptly leaves the meeting.

Question One

What is the team's best response?

A. Suggest that the administrator look for a new medical director.

B. Arrange for a team member to talk with Jay.

C. Call one of Jay's partners and report his uncharacteristic behavior.

D. Ignore Jay's behavior and hope he calms down.

Correct Response and Analysis

The correct response is B. A respected team colleague might be able to help Jay to voice his concerns and participate in focused problem solving. Response A is incorrect because it is premature and makes a scapegoat of Jay. C is incorrect because the team should first try to resolve its problems internally, and D is incorrect because ignoring the situation is unlikely to resolve the very real problems that confront both Jay and the program.

The Case Continues

Walter, the program's chaplain, has been Jay's friend for some time, so the team asks him to contact Jay. Walter agrees, calls Jay at the office, and asks to meet with him over lunch. During lunch, Walter expresses his concern and asks Jay to talk about what is going on in his life. At first Jay is reluctant because he is somewhat embarrassed about his outburst at the meeting, but with encouragement from Walter, he describes the numerous stressors in his life. He talks about his seeming inability to "fix things" at home, at the office, or at the hospice. He also talks about his increasing feelings of anger and the guilt he feels for exhibiting impatience.

Walter acknowledges that Jay is in a very tough spot, then politely suggests that Jay might benefit from information on stress management, which might help him to cope better with team members. Walter explores Jay's willingness to obtain counseling, but Jay is very resistant. Walter asks Jay about activities that have helped him to cope with stress in the past. Jay used to ride his bicycle and jog regularly, but now he rarely has time to do either. When Walter asks Jay about vacations, Jay says he and his wife have been too busy to take any vacation during the past year.

Question Two

What are the three best courses of action for Walter to take?

A. Insist that Jay begin counseling.

B. Encourage Jay to schedule time for exercise.

C. Encourage Jay to schedule time for a vacation.

D. Encourage Jay to make amends with the nurse and become actively involved with the team in analyzing problems and developing solutions

Correct Responses and Analysis

The correct responses are B, C, and D. Exercise and time for relaxation are likely to help Jay to cope with a very stressful set of circumstances, regain his sense of perspective, and enhance his sense of competence and control. Making amends with the nurse will improve team functioning, and a careful analysis of the program's current problems is likely to shed some light on possible solutions. Response A is incorrect at this time because Jay is unlikely to comply with or benefit from an intervention that he has refused.

The Case Concludes

Walter suggests that lack of exercise may be contributing to Jay's difficulties in coping with stress. He recommends that Jay and Katherine make a commitment to exercise three times a week for 30 minutes. Walter also points out that taking a vacation may be the most helpful thing that Jay can do for the program, his practice, and his family. Jay finally smiles.

Jay recalls a time when his partner was experiencing a lot of distress. Jay suggested counseling and antidepressant medication, which helped the partner a lot. Walter politely points out the similarities between the partner's position then and Jay's position now, and reminds Jay about the discussion on burnout prevention in the Academy's UNIPAC series. Jay acknowledges the difficulties that he is having and says that he will think about Walter's suggestions.

That afternoon, Jay visits with the patient whose symptoms were unrelieved over the weekend, orders additional medication changes, and is gratified when the patient's symptoms begin to abate.

That evening, Jay and his wife talk about making time for exercise and a vacation. They commit to exercising three times a week and agree on times that will respect the family's needs. Jay agrees to schedule time to care for their son while Katherine exercises or rests. Then they agree to take a vacation during Katherine's spring break, three weeks away. The next day Jay talks with his partners and schedules a week's vacation. Jay and his partners also agree to focus on resolving their differences with the managed-care company. Jay makes amends with the hospice nurse by acknowledging the difficulties that she is facing and revealing some of his own personal difficulties.

Jay calls the hospice administrator and requests a meeting with the management team after he returns from vacation. He recommends that the team analyze the challenges that the program is facing and develop specific coping strategies. He also suggests that the management team analyze staff/patient ratios, review the charts of patients whose symptoms are not adequately controlled within an agreed-upon time, analyze physician referral patterns, and summarize the results of satisfaction surveys completed by patients, families, and physicians to track trends in complaints. The administrator agrees, and the meeting is scheduled.

During the next week, Jay and his partners complete their negotiations with the managed-care company and sign the contracts.

By reducing the stressors in his life and using previously successful coping techniques, including physical exercise, Jay begins to feel better. He vows to initiate counseling if the vacation and continued physical exercise don't bring him considerable relief. Katherine writes a "thank you" note to Walter.

Pretest Correct Answers

1. A	20. C
2. B	21. B
3. D	22. D
4. A	23. D
5. C	24. A
6. C	25. A
7. B	26. B
8. D	27. B
9. A	28. B
10. C	29. C
11. A	30. A
12. B	31. D
13. D	32. D
14. D	33. A
15. A	34. D
16. B	35. C
17. D	36. D
18. C	37. B
19. D	38. A

Posttest

Read each item and circle the **one** correct response to each item on the detachable answer sheet at the back of the book.

1. **All the following statements about communication skills are true *except* which one?**

   A. When training to improve nonverbal communication skills, audiotapes are more effective than visual aides.

   B. Videotaping interactions with simulated patients and receiving feedback from experienced facilitators are effective means for improving communication skills.

   C. Beneficial behavior changes are most likely to occur when skills training is coupled with exercises that enhance personal growth and awareness.

   D. Careful discipline is required to develop reliable skills in interviewing and in understanding the meaning of the patient's communications.

2. **Strategies for managing stress include all the following *except* which one?**

   A. Developing professional skills and setting realistic goals

   B. Making independent decisions and relying on informal decision-making protocols

   C. Acknowledging life's imperfections and the impossibility of guaranteeing a perfect outcome for every patient and family

   D. Exercising, participating in outside activities for their intrinsic enjoyment, and setting limits on involvement with professional and civic organizations

3. **All the following statements about team member roles are true *except* which one?**

   A. Role ambiguity, role conflict, and role overload impede individual and team performance.

   B. Role ambiguity occurs when roles and expectations are poorly defined and inadequately communicated.

   C. Role conflict can be alleviated by listing all the tasks associated with each role and discussing areas of role overlap.

   D. Role overload is rarely associated with unrealistic personal expectations regarding job performance or crises in the personal lives of team members.

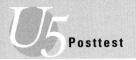

4. **Which of the following statements about confidentiality is correct?**

   A. Team members are required to share all patient and family information with other members of the team.

   B. Confidentiality is breached when a team member shares confidential information without the patient's permission.

   C. Confidentiality is an absolute obligation that must always be observed.

   D. Trying to negotiate the amount of confidential information that can be shared with other team members is inappropriate behavior.

5. **Which of the following statements about effective negotiation is correct?**

   A. It clarifies the participants' views.

   B. It focuses primarily on long-term goals.

   C. It encourages rapid identification of a solution.

   D. It discourages emphasis on each participant's dignity and self-esteem.

6. **When terminally ill patients ask for more information about how much time they have left to live, which of the following is the most appropriate response?**

   A. I would guess about _____ (fill in a specific number of days, weeks, or months).

   B. There is really no point in trying to guess; everyone is different.

   C. There is always a lot of uncertainty when estimating length of life because people generally live longer or shorter than an average. Based on the medical indications and your situation, you are likely to live about ____ (fill in a range of estimated number of days, weeks, months, e.g., several weeks and maybe as much as a few months).

   D. I think such information would depress you and destroy all of your hope, so I prefer not to talk about it.

7. **All the following statements about discussing prognosis are true except which one?**

   A. Patients rarely want much information about prognosis.

   B. A precise estimate of life expectancy may become a fixed sentence in the patient's mind.

C. When patients request information about prognosis, physicians should provide estimates that are as accurate as possible.

D. Physicians should encourage patients to complete the developmental tasks of the dying.

8. **Which of the following statements is correct?**

A. Physicians tend to interrupt their patients within the first 18 seconds of an interview.

B. Minimal leads, such as "Uh-huh," "Umm," and "Ah," are ineffective listening techniques.

C. Confrontation is an inappropriate technique in palliative care settings.

D. The following is an example of repetition: "What is going on when you are not feeling good?"

9. **All the following statements are true *except* which one?**

A. There is little correlation between the likelihood of a medical malpractice suit and a physician's ability to communicate effectively.

B. A physician's ability to communicate effectively with patients is affected by the physician's own intrapersonal communication.

C. Effective communication with patients during the history-taking process contributes more information about diagnosis than laboratory tests.

D. Therapeutic communication is important, even when interacting with comatose patients.

10. **Signs and symptoms of physician stress overload include all the following *except* which one?**

A. Anger, irritability, frustration, and tiredness out of proportion to the work that is being done

B. Overconscientiousness, impaired perspective, and preoccupation with patients

C. Distancing, intellectualization, and loss of sense of humor

D. Ability to establish a satisfying balance between professional and home responsibilities

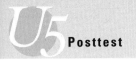

11. **All the following statements about effective teams are true *except* which one?**

    A. Effective teams expect team members to assertively represent their discipline's current practice standards.

    B. Effective teams recognize and honor the expertise of each team member and carefully evaluate how each discipline can contribute to the patient's and family's well-being.

    C. Effective teams expect individual and collective accountability for developing interventions and following through.

    D. Effective teams rely on the talents of one experienced team member to provide leadership.

12. **All the following statements about denial are true *except* which one?**

    A. Denial is a commonly used unconscious response for coping with the implications of a terminal illness; it usually waxes and wanes throughout the course of the terminal illness.

    B. Whenever possible, physicians and other healthcare professionals should break down a patient's denial so that reality can be confronted more effectively.

    C. A family's insistence on withholding information from the patient is likely to result from the family members' own death-related fears.

    D. Instead of acquiescing with a family's demand to withhold information, physicians should help family members to explore their concerns, normalize their fears, and provide education.

13. **When physicians participate in family conferences, which of the following behaviors is least appropriate?**

    A. Exhibiting primary loyalty to the patient

    B. Correcting misconceptions about diagnosis and treatments

    C. Acknowledging the patient's and family's fears, grief, and guilt

    D. Helping patients and families to identify strengths and set realistic short-term goals

14. **When terminally ill patients first ask if they are dying, which of the following is most likely to be an appropriate response?**

    A. There is no need to talk about dying now. I'll let you know when the time comes to worry.

B. It's hard to say; everyone is terminal. We're all dying.

C. Yes. You probably have no more than _____ (fill in the correct number of days, weeks, or months) left to live.

D. Based on the medical evidence, your situation does look very serious. What are some of your main concerns about dying?

15. When patients respond emotionally to bad news, which of the following statements is true?

A. As soon as patients or family members start to cry, hand them a facial tissue.

B. When patients respond with anger, the most important first step is to correct factual misconceptions.

C. After emotions have cooled, trying to use a problem-solving approach will escalate the patient's anger.

D. Anger is usually based on displaced fear and/or feelings of being ignored and devalued.

16. All the following statements about communication techniques, such as listening, acknowledging, clarifying, reassuring, and validating, are true *except* which one?

A. They can serve as powerful treatment interventions.

B. They can influence a patient's expectations.

C. They can affect the patient's emotional and physical well-being.

D. They encourage patients to focus exclusively on physical symptoms.

17. All the following statements are true *except* which one?

A. Honest communication increases a patient's and family's sense of control and self-worth.

B. For terminally ill patients, a sense of being heard may be the most effective healing agent.

C. Because unrelieved symptoms and stress interfere with a patient's ability to hear and retain information, physicians should focus on alleviating distressing symptoms, establishing a therapeutic relationship, and repeating information as often as needed.

D. Poor communication skills may interfere with a physician's ability to perform an adequate history, but they have little impact on the patient's overall sense of suffering.

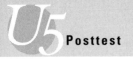

18. **All the following statements about a physician's role on the interdisciplinary team are correct *except* which one?**

    A. Attending physicians should provide the admitting diagnosis and prognosis, order medications and treatments, make inpatient and home care visits when needed, provide medical management of conditions unrelated to the terminal illness, and designate an emergency on-call physician.

    B. Hospice medical directors should confirm the terminal diagnosis, determine the medical appropriateness of treatment options and goals, participate in team meetings, consult with attending physicians when necessary, and evaluate patients in home or inpatient settings as needed.

    C. Hospice medical directors should serve as interdisciplinary team leaders, provide leadership during most family conferences, and approve medical, social, spiritual, and psychological interventions.

    D. Hospice medical directors must be doctors of medicine or osteopathy with a current license to practice and to prescribe scheduled drugs.

19. **All the following statements about interdisciplinary teamwork are true *except* which one?**

    A. The process of decision making is more efficient and takes less time.

    B. More effort is needed to communicate effectively and to maintain effective team functioning.

    C. Varied professional perspectives may result in comprehensive interventions that meet a patient's physical, social, emotional, and spiritual needs.

    D. Shared responsibility may result in a lack of individual responsibility or accountability.

20. **Which of the following statements about family conferences is correct?**

    A. Effective physicians are able to resolve the family's long-standing problems.

    B. When counseling with patients and families, effective physicians involve other team members, such as a hospice/palliative care nurse, social worker, or chaplain.

    C. Effective physicians can control the outcome of family conferences.

    D. Physicians are responsible for the choices made by patients and family members.

21. **A family system's response to terminal illness is likely to be affected by which of the following?**

    A. The patient's roles in the family

    B. The family system's rules regarding communication and interaction with the outside world

    C. The ability of remaining family members to perform essential tasks

    D. All the above

22. **All the following statements about sharing bad news are true *except* which one?**

    A. Use simple, everyday language, i.e., no medical jargon or euphemisms.

    B. Fire "warning shots" to indicate that the situation is worse than expected, e.g., "I'm afraid your symptoms indicate that the illness is taking a turn for the worse."

    C. The most important factor is determining precisely how much information a referring physician has shared with the patient about diagnosis and prognosis.

    D. Repeat information as often as needed.

23. **When sharing bad news, which of the following statements is correct?**

    A. Avoid statements or inquiries that are likely to elicit painful emotions on the part of the patient or family.

    B. Use medical vocabulary so that patients and families can learn to speak intelligently about the patient's condition.

    C. First give a brief, rapid summary of the patient's diagnosis and prognosis, then go back over the information more slowly.

    D. When patients no longer appear to be listening, bring the interview to a close and reschedule a follow-up after patients and families have had time to assimilate the news.

24. **In most situations, which of the following nonverbal behaviors is least likely to communicate empathy?**

    A. Sitting down so the physician's eyes are slightly lower than the patient's

    B. Sitting very close to the patient, about 12 to 18 inches

    C. Sitting about 20 to 36 inches from the patient

    D. Sitting in a relaxed position and leaning toward the patient

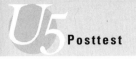

25. **A patient's reluctance to discuss diagnosis and prognosis is likely to result from all the following *except* which one?**

    A. A need to periodically deny the existence of a life-threatening condition

    B. The widespread belief among patients that information about diagnosis and prognosis will do them harm

    C. The desire to protect themselves, their family members, and their physicians from the distressing emotions that often accompany discussions of poor prognosis

    D. Subtle, nonverbal cues from the physician indicating that such discussions are unwelcome

26. **Characteristics of effective team members include which of the following?**

    A. Professional competence and excellent communication skills

    B. Patience, flexibility, and tolerance of ambiguity

    C. Ability to set personal limits and to take responsibility for actions

    D. All the above

27. **All the following statements about the interdisciplinary team approach to care are true *except* which one?**

    A. The Medicare Hospice Benefit requires the use of a core team consisting of a physician, a registered nurse, a social worker, and a pastoral or other counselor.

    B. The Medicare Hospice Benefit requires that core members of the team meet at least once every 2 weeks to review each patient's status and care plan.

    C. The team leader bears final responsibility for the team's decisions and has final authority to implement treatment options.

    D. The team is responsible for developing an individualized interdisciplinary plan of care that meets the physical, emotional, social, and spiritual needs of each patient.

28. **Which of the following statements is correct?**

    A. Members of enmeshed families rarely experience significant grief-related problems because the family system's beliefs encourage individuals to develop identities apart from the family.

    B. Functional enmeshment is particularly inappropriate when families are coping with a patient's terminal illness.

UNIPAC Five: Caring for the Terminally Ill—Communication and the Physician's Role on the Interdisciplinary Team

C. Members of open family systems rarely experience significant stress during a patient's terminal illness.

D. Members of open family systems are more likely to view change as inevitable and to use direct communication when talking about problems.

29. **When sharing bad news, which of the following statements is true?**

A. Physicians should wear white coats to emphasize their professional knowledge and authority.

B. Televisions and radios should be left on to provide welcome distractions from the bad news.

C. Physicians should provide reassurance by emphasizing that "everything is going to be fine."

D. Physicians should always sit down when sharing bad news.

30. **When physicians communicate bad news, patients prefer all the following *except* which one?**

A. Direct, empathic communication that includes information about diagnosis

B. High levels of sustained optimism and continued emphasis on the positive aspects of the situation

C. Information about prognosis and how it is likely to affect their plans for the future

D. Inclusion of a family member or friend when bad news is shared.

31. **Which the following statements about communications is correct?**

A. To ensure effective communication with patients, most physicians can easily switch from "medical" language to "everyday" language.

B. When dying patients have limited English language skills, physicians can rely on the patient's friends and/or family members to provide reliable interpretation.

C. When physicians engage in meaningful communication and try to understand a patient's point of view, their own long-held beliefs may be challenged by the patient's beliefs and experiences.

D. Most physicians, nurses, and patients understand commonly used medical and psychological terms.

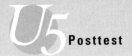
32. **Which of the following statements is true?**

    A. Most patients believe that information about their diagnosis and prognosis benefits them, even when the news is bad.

    B. The manner in which bad news about a diagnosis is communicated is less important than the inclusion of complete descriptions of all test results.

    C. Experienced, skilled physicians can easily determine how much information patients want about diagnosis and prognosis.

    D. When a physician's nonverbal cues contradict a verbal message, patients are much more likely to believe the physician's verbal statements.

33. **All the following statements are true *except* which one?**

    A. A patient's most basic needs are the need to know and understand the diagnosis and prognosis and the need to feel known and understood by the physician.

    B. When physicians interact with patients, just the act of sitting down increases patient satisfaction.

    C. A lighthearted approach to terminal illness increases patient satisfaction.

    D. Patient satisfaction depends more on the perception of a physician's emotional support and adequate sharing of information than on the amount of time that the physician actually spends with patients.

34. **All the following statements are true *except* which one?**

    A. To help terminally ill patients to regain a sense of perspective, physicians should tell jokes and try to be funny.

    B. Patients sometimes use humor as a powerful intervention for coping with loss.

    C. Humor requires the ability to step back from a situation and recognize its paradoxical qualities.

    D. Sensitivity and intuition are critical when using humor in the palliative care setting.

35. **All the following statements about empathy are true *except* which one?**

    A. Empathy refers to the ability to identify a patient's emotions.

    B. Empathy refers to the ability to hear the unspoken questions and messages that lie underneath a patient's words.

C. Empathic response requires physical contact, such as a hug or a pat on the back.

D. Empathy refers to the ability to recognize when listening is a more appropriate intervention than ordering additional medications or procedures.

36. **All the following statements about sharing bad news are true *except* which one?**

   A. Communication should be an ongoing event, and the pace should be determined by the patient's personality and desire to know more.

   B. Patients are more interested in diagnosis and treatment plans than in the illness's likely impact on themselves and their family members.

   C. Physicians and nurses consistently underestimate the type and amount of information that patients want to know.

   D. Most patients know that they are dying, so avoiding discussion of their prognosis is likely to increase their sense of isolation.

37. **After sharing bad news about diagnosis and prognosis, which of the following is the least appropriate role for a physician?**

   A. Help patients and families to identify specific problems and distinguish those that are fixable from those that are not.

   B. Leave patients and families alone so that they can devise their own situation-specific solutions for coping.

   C. Help patients and families to identify successful coping strategies and past and current sources of support.

   D. Remind patients and family members that the entire team will be available to answers questions, provide support, and help to resolve problems.

38. **Which of the following statements about conflict resolution is correct?**

   A. Effective facilitators welcome the existence of conflict and view it as an opportunity for positive change.

   B. Effective facilitators encourage participants to address all areas of conflict.

   C. Effective facilitators concentrate more on long-term goals than on short-term goals.

   D. Effective facilitators encourage participants to chose several solutions and implement all of them.

References

[1] Katz J. *The Silent World of Doctor and Patient.* New York: The Free Press; 1984.

[2] Buckman R. Communication in palliative care: a practical guide. In: Doyle D, Hanks GWC, MacDonald N, eds. *Oxford Textbook of Palliative Medicine.* New York: Oxford University Press; 1993:47–61.

[3] Buckman R. *How to Break Bad News: A Guide for Health Care Professionals.* Baltimore, Md: Johns Hopkins University Press; 1992.

[4] Irwin WG, McClelland R, Love AHG. Communication skills training for medical students: an integrated approach. *Med Edu.* 1989;23:387.

[5] Roter DL, Hall JA. Doctors Talking with Patients, Patients Talking with Doctors. Auburn House. Westport, Conn. 1992. Cited by: Ong LML, DeHaes JCJM, Hoos AM, Lammes FB. Doctor–patient communication: a review of the literature. *Soc Sci Med.* 1995;40(7):903–918.

[6] Stagno SJ, Zhukovsky DS, Walsh D. Bioethics: communication and decision-making in advanced disease. *Semin Oncol.* 2000;27(1):94–100.

[7] Silveira MJ, DiPiero A, Gerrity MS, Feudtner C. Patients' knowledge of options at the end of life: ignorance in the face of death. *JAMA.* 2000;284(19):2483–2488.

[8] Buckman R. Communication in palliative care: a practical guide. In: Doyle D, Hanks GWC, MacDonald N, eds. *Oxford Textbook of Palliative Medicine*, 2nd ed. New York: Oxford University Press; 1998:141–156.

[9] Ong LML, DeHaes JCJM, Hoos AM, Lammes FB. Doctor–patient communication: a review of the literature. *Soc Sci Med.* 1995;40(7):903–918.

[10] Jonsen AR, Siegler M, Winslade WJ. *Clinical Ethics: A Practical Approach to Ethical Decisions in Clinical Medicine.* New York: Macmillan;1982.

[11] Charon R. Narrative medicine: a model for empathy, reflection, profession, and trust. *JAMA.* 2001;286(15):1897–1902.

[12] Detmar SB, Muller MJ, Wever LD, Schornagel JH, Aaronson NK. The patient-physician relationship. Patient-physician communication during outpatient palliative treatment visits: an observational study. *JAMA.* 2001;285(10):1351–1357.

[13] Quill TE. Perspective on care at the close of life. Initiating end-of-life discussions with seriously ill patients: addressing the "elephant in the room." *JAMA.* 2000;284(19):2502–2507.

[14] Cohen-Cole SA. *The Medical Interview: The Three Function Approach.* Boston: Mosby Year Book; 1991.

[15] Kramer P. Doctors discuss how to break bad news. *ASCO Daily News.* 1998;1(4):8–9. Cited in: Baile WF, Kudelka AP, Beale EA, Glober GA, Myers EG, Greisinger AJ, Bast RC, Goldstein MG, Novack D, Lenzi R. Communication skills training in oncology: description and preliminary outcomes of workshops on breaking bad news and managing patient reactions to illness. *Cancer.* 1999;86(5):887–897.

[16] Johnston M. Communicating the diagnosis of motor neurone disease. *Palliat Med.* 1996;10:23–34.

[17] Byock IR. The nature of suffering and the nature of opportunity at the end of life. *Clin Geriatr Med.* 1996;12(2):237–252.

[18] Billings JA, Stoeckle JD. *The Clinical Encounter: A Guide to the Medical Interview and Case Presentation.* Chicago: Year Book Medical Publishers; 1989.

AAHPM

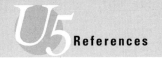
[19]Doyle D. Have we looked beyond the physical and psychosocial? Presented at the International Hospice Institute Seventh Annual Symposium; July 10–14, 1991: Washington, D.C.

[20]Adson MA. An endangered ethic—the capacity for caring. *Mayo Clin Proc*. 1995;70:495–500.

[21]Schweizer H. To give suffering a language. *Lit Med*. 1995;14(2):210–221.

[22]Doukas DJ, Brody H. Care at the twilight: ethics and end-of-life care. *Am Fam Physician*. 1995;52(5):94.

[23]Winslow R. Sometimes, talk is the best medicine. For physicians, communication may avert suits. *Wall Street Journal*, October 5, 1989, p. B1.

[24]Levinson W, Roter DL, Mullooly JP, Dull VT, Frankel RM. Physician–patient communication. The relationship with malpractice claims among primary care physicians and surgeons. *JAMA*. 1997;277(7):553–559.

[25]Eisenberg L. Medicine—molecular, monetary, or more than both? *JAMA*. 1995;274(4):331–334.

[26]Hickson GB, Calyton EW, Entmann SS, et al. Obstetricians' prior malpractice experience and patients' satisfaction with care. *JAMA*. 1994;272:1593–1587. Cited by: Eisenberg L. Medicine—molecular, monetary, or more than both? *JAMA*. 1995;274(4):331–334.

[27]Entman SS, Glass CA, Hickson GB, Githens PB, Whetten-Goldstein K, Sloan FA. The relationship between malpractice claims history and subsequent obstetric care. *JAMA*. 1994;272:1588–1591. Cited by: Eisenberg L. Medicine—molecular, monetary, or more than both? *JAMA*. 1995;274(4):331–334.

[28]Hampton JR, Harrison MJG, Mitchell JRA, Pritchard JS, Seymour C. Relative contributions of history-taking, physical examination, and laboratory investigation to diagnosis and management of medical outpatients. *Br Med J*. 1975;1486–1489. Cited by: Eisenberg L. Medicine—molecular, monetary, or more than both? *JAMA*. 1995;274(4):331–334.

[29]Peterson MC, Holbrook JH, Hales DV, Smith NL. Staker LV. Contributions of the history of physical examination, and laboratory investigation in making medical diagnoses. *West J Med*. 1992;156:163–165. Cited by: Eisenberg L. Medicine—molecular, monetary, or more than both? *JAMA*. 1995;274(4):331–334.

[30]Chaitchik S, Kreitler S, Shaked S, Schwartz I, Rosin R. Doctor–patient communication in a cancer ward. *J Cancer Edu*. 1992;7:41. Cited in: Ong LML, DeHaes JCJM, Hoos AM, Lammes FB. Doctor–patient communication: a review of the literature. *Soc Sci Med*. 1995;40(7):903–918.

[31]Holland JC, Almanza J. Giving bad news: is there a kinder, gentler way? *Cancer*. 1999;86(5):738–740.

[32]Lipson JG, Dibble SL, Minarik PA. *Culture and Nursing Care: A Pocket Guide*. School of Nursing, University of California. San Francisco: UCSF Nursing Press; 1996.

[33]Honeybun J, Johnston M, Tookman A. The impact of a death on fellow hospice patients. *Br J Med Psychol*. 1992;65:67–72. Cited by: Johnston M, Earll L, Mitchell E, Morrison V, Wright S. Communicating the diagnosis of motor neurone disease. *Palliat Med*. 1996;10:23–34.

[34]Bruera E, Neumann CM, Mazzocato C, Stiefel F, Sala R. Attitudes and beliefs of palliative care physicians regarding communication with terminally ill cancer patients. *Palliat Med*. 2000;14(4):287–298.

[35]Vanchieri C. Cultural gaps leave patients angry, doctors confused. *Hospice*. 1996;7(3):7–8. Published by the National Hospice Institute. Reprinted from: *J Natl Cancer Inst*. 1995;87(21).

[36]Fitch MI. How much should I say to whom? *J Palliat Care*. 1994;10(3):90–100.

[37]Rogers CR, Roethlisberger FJ. Barriers and gateways to communication. *Harvard Business Rev*. November–December, 1991:105–111.

[38]Feifel H. Toward death: a psychological perspective. In: Schneidmen ES, ed. *Death: Current Perspectives.* Palo Alto, Calif.: Mayfield Publishing Co. 1976. Cited by: Fallowfield L. Giving sad and bad news. *Lancet.* 1993;341:476–478.

[39]Maguire P, Faulkner A. How to do it: improve the counseling skills of doctors and nurses in cancer care. *Br Med J.* 1988;297:847–849. Cited by: Buckman R. Communication in palliative care: a practical guide. In: Doyle D, Hanks GWC, MacDonald N, eds. *Oxford Textbook of Palliative Medicine.* New York: Oxford University Press; 1993:47–61.

[40]SUPPORT. The SUPPORT clinical investigators. A controlled trial to improve care for seriously ill hospitalized patients. *JAMA.* 1995;274:1591–1598.

[41]White WL, Kunz C, Hogan J. Communication skills. In: *Hospice Education Program for Nurses.* US DHHS Publication No. HRA 81–27. 1981.

[42]Bourhis RY, Roth S, MacQueen G. Communication in the hospital setting: a survey of medical and everyday language use amongst patients, nurses, and doctors. *Soc Sci Med.* 1989;28:339.

[43]Woloshin S, Bickell NA, Schwartz LM, Gany F, Welch HG. Language barriers in medicine in the United States. *JAMA.* 1995;273(9):724–728.

[44]Putsch RW. Cross-cultural communication: the special case of interpreters in health care. *JAMA.* 1985;254(23):3344–3348.

[45]Hadlow J, Pitts M. The understanding of common health terms by doctors, nurses and patients. *Soc. Sci. Med.* 1991;32:193. Cited by: Ong LML, DeHaes JCJM, Hoos AM, Lammes FB. Doctor–patient communication: a review of the literature. *Soc Sci Med.* 1995;40(7):903–918.

[46]Bensing JM. Doctor–patient communication and the quality of care. An observation study into affective and instrumental behavior in general practice. Dissertation. NIVEL. Utrecht, 1991. Cited by: Ong LML, DeHaes JCJM, Hoos AM, Lammes FB. Doctor–patient communication: a review of the literature. *Soc Sci Med.* 1995;40(7):903–918.

[47]Friedman HS. Non-verbal communications between patients and medical practitioners. *J Soc Issues.* 1979;35:82.

[48]Lumsden G, Lumsden D. *Communicating in Groups and Teams.* 2nd ed. New York: Wadsworth; 1996.

[49]Hamilton C, Parker C. *Communicating for Results: A Guide for Business and the Professions.* 4th ed. Belmont, Calif: Wadsworth; 1993.

[50]Quill TE. Recognizing and adjusting to barriers in doctor–patient communication. *Ann Intern Med.* 1989;111(1):51–57.

[51]Delbanco TL. Enriching the doctor–patient relationship by inviting the patient's perspective. *Ann Intern Med.* 1992;116(5):415–418.

[52]Miller RJ. Communication and truth telling in terminal illness. Presented at: Principles and Practice of Hospice Medicine, Unit I: Patient Care in a Hospice Setting. Academy of Hospice Physicians. April 2–5, 1992; Philadelphia, Pa.

[53]Williamson DS, Noel ML. Systemic family medicine: an evolving concept. In: Rakel RE, ed. *Textbook of Family Practice.* 4th ed. Philadelphia: WB Saunders; 1990:61–79.

[54]Lunn L. Spiritual concerns in palliation. In: Saunders C, Sykes N, eds. *Management of Terminal Malignancies.* 3rd ed. Boston: Edward Arnold; 1993.

[55]Ptacek JT, Eberhardt T. Breaking bad news. *JAMA.* 1996;276(6):496–502.

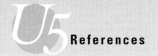
[56]Fry WF. The physiologic effects of humor, mirth, and laughter. *JAMA*. 1992;267(13):1857–1858.

[57]Wooten P. Humor: an antidote for stress. *Holistic Nurs Pract*. 1996;10(2): 49–56.

[58]Dean RA. Humor and laughter in palliative care. *J Palliat Care*. 1997;13(1):34–39.

[59]Goodman JB. Laughing matters: taking your job seriously and yourself lightly. *JAMA*. 1992;267(13):1858.

[60]Perrino AF. *Holyquest: The Search for Wholeness*. Carmel, Calif.: Sunflower Ink; 1988.

[61]Herth K. Fostering hope in terminally ill people. *J Advan Nurs*. 1990;15:1250–1259.

[62]Fletcher CM. Communication in medicine. (*Rock Carling Monograph*). London: Nuffield Provincial Hospital Trust, 1973. Quoted by: Johnston M, Earll L, Mitchell E, Morrison V, Wright S. Communicating the diagnosis of motor neurone disease. *Palliat Med*. 1996;10:23–34.

[63]Bor R, Miller R, Goldman E, Scher I. The meaning of bad news in HIV disease: counseling about dreaded issues revisited. *Counsel Psychol Q*. 1993;6:69–80. Quoted by: Ptacek JT, Eberhardt TL. Breaking bad news: a review of the literature. *JAMA*. 1996;276(6):496–502.

[64]Johnston M, Earll L, Mitchell E, Morrison V, Wright S. Communicating the diagnosis of motor neurone disease. *Palliat Med*. 1996;10:23–34.

[65]Robinson. *Multiple Sclerosis*. London: Routledge; 1988. Cited by: Johnston M, Earll L, Mitchell E, Morrison V, Wright S. Communicating the diagnosis of motor neurone disease. *Palliat Med*. 1996;10:23–34.

[66]von Gunten CF. Discussing hospice care. *J Clin Oncol*. 2000;20(5):

[67]Foley, K. A 44–year-old woman with severe pain at the end of life. *JAMA*. 1999;281(20):1937–1945.

[68]von Gunten CF, Ferris FD, Emanuel LL. Ensuring competency in end-of-life care: communication and relational skills. *JAMA*. 2000;284(23):3051–3057.

[69]Hamilton C, Parker C. *Communicating for Results: A Guide for Business and the Professions*. 4th ed. Belmont, Calif.: Wadsworth; 1993.

[70]Waitzkin H. Doctor–patient communication. Clinical implications of social scientific research. *JAMA*. 1984;252:2441. Cited by: Ong LML, DeHaes JCJM, Hoos AM, Lammes FB. Doctor–patient communication: a review of the literature. *Soc Sci Med*. 1995;40(7):903–918.

[71]Fletcher WS. Doctor, am I terminal? *Am J Surg*. 1992;163:460–462.

[72]Byock I. *Dying Well: The Prospect for Growth at the End of Life*. New York: Riverhead Books; 1997.

[73]Schonwetter RS, Teasdale TA, Luchi RJ, Storey P. Estimation of survival time in terminal cancer patients: an impedance to hospice admissions? *Hospice J*. 1990;6(4):65–79.

[74]Fallowfield L. Giving sad and bad news. *Lancet*. 1993;341:476–478.

[75]Beasley NW, Wheby MS, Pruett TL. Medical center hour: breaking the bad news. *Va Med Q*. 1993;120:90–93. Cited by: Ptacek JT, Eberhardt TL. Breaking bad news: a review of the literature. *JAMA*. 1996;276(6):496–502.

[76]Minuchin S. *Families and Family Therapy*. London: Tavistock Publications. 1974. Cited by: White WL, Kunz C, Hogan J. Communication skills. In: *Hospice Education Program for Nurses*. US DHHS Publication No. HRA 81–27. 1981.

[77]Satir V. *The New Peoplemaking*. Palo Alto, Calif.: Science and Behavior Books; 1988.

[78]Huygen FJA. *Family Medicine: The Medical Life History of Families*. New York: Brunner/Mazel, Inc.;

1982:147–148. Cited by: Willamson DS, Noel ML. Systemic family medicine: an evolving concept. In: Rakel RE. *Textbook of Family Medicine*. 4th ed. Philadelphia: WB Saunders; 1990:61–79.

[79]Glenn ML. *Collaborative Health Care: A Family-Oriented Model*. New York: Praeger; 1987. Cited by: Willamson DS, Noel ML. Systemic family medicine: an evolving concept. In: Rakel RE. *Textbook of Family Medicine*. 4th ed. Philadelphia: WB Saunders; 1990:61–79.

[80]Ajemian I. The interdisciplinary team. In: Doyle D, Hanks GWC, MacDonald N, eds. *Oxford Textbook of Palliative Medicine*. New York: Oxford University Press; 1993:17–29.

[81]Fisher R, Ury W. *Getting to Yes: Negotiating Agreement Without Giving In*. Boston: Houghton-Mifflin; 1981.

[82]Alexander DA. Psychological/social research. In: Doyle D, Hanks GWC, MacDonald N, eds. *Oxford Textbook of Palliative Medicine*. New York: Oxford University Press;1993:92–96.

[83]Wilkinson J. Ethical issues in palliative care. In: Doyle D, Hanks GWC, MacDonald N, eds. *Oxford Textbook of Palliative Medicine*. New York: Oxford University Press; 1993:495–504.

[84]Kircher P. *Love Is the Link*. Burdette, N.Y.: Larson Publishers; 1995.

[85]Callanan-Pflaum M, Kelley P. *Final Gifts*. New York: Poseidon Press; 1992.

[86]Katzenbach JR, Smith DK. The discipline of teams. *Harvard Business Rev*. 1993;March/April:111–120.

[87]Mount BM. Dealing with our losses. *J Clin Oncol*. 1986;4(7):1127–1134.

[88]Cassell EJ. The nature of suffering and the goals of medicine. *N Engl J Med*. 1982;306:639–645.

[89]Health Care Finance Administration. Federal Regulations for a Medicare Hospice Program. Regulation Part 418.

[90]National Hospice Organization. *Standards of a Hospice Program of Care*. Arlington, Va.: National Hospice Organization; 1993.

[91]Drinka TJK. Applying learning from self-directed work teams in business to curriculum development. *Educ Gerontol*. 1996;22:433–450.

[92]Zeiss AM, Steffen AM. Interdisciplinary health care teams: the basic unit of geriatric care. In: Carstensen LL, Edelstein BA, Dornbrand L, eds. *The Practical Handbook of Clinical Gerontology*. Thousand Oaks, Calif.: Sage Publishing; 1996.

[93]Lattanzi-Licht M. The hospice team: the wonder, worries and work. *The Hospice Professional*. National Hospice Organization: Arlington, Va.: Autumn 1996.

[94]Drinka TJK. Interdisciplinary geriatric teams: approaches to conflict as indicators of potential to model teamwork. *Educ. Gerontol*. 1994;20:87–103.

[95]Juliá, MC, Thompson A. Essential elements of interprofessional teamwork. In: Casto RM, Juliá, MC, Platt LJ, Harbaugh GL, Waugaman WR, Thompson A, Jost TS, Bope ET, Williams T, Lee DB, eds. *Interprofessional Care and Collaborative Practice*. Pacific Grove, Calif.: Brooks/Cole Publishing; 1994:43–57.

[96]Randall F, Downie RS. *Palliative Care Ethics*. Oxford: Oxford Medical Publications; 1996:40–59.

[97]West T. The interdisciplinary hospice team. Presented at Seventh International Congress on Care of the Terminally Ill. Montreal; September, 1990. Cited by: Ajemian I. The interdisciplinary team. In: Doyle D, Hanks GWC, MacDonald N, eds. *Oxford Textbook of Palliative Medicine*. New York: Oxford University Press; 1993:17–29.

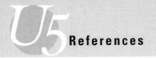

[98]Lowe JI, Herranen M. Interdisciplinary team. In: *Hospice Education Program for Nurses*. Washington, D.C.: U.S. Department of Health and Human Services Publication No. HRA 81–27; 1981:1047–1048.

[99]Johnson DW, Johnson FP. *Joining Together: Group Theory and Group Skills*. Englewood Cliffs, N.J.: Prentice Hall; 1975:109. Cited by: Juliá, MC, Thompson A. Essential elements of interprofessional teamwork. In: Casto RM, Juliá, MC, Platt LJ, Harbaugh GL, Waugaman WR, Thompson A, Jost TS, Bope ET, Williams T, Lee DB, eds. *Interprofessional Care and Collaborative Practice*. Pacific Grove, Calif.: Brooks/Cole Publishing; 1994:43–57.

[100]Lefton RE. The eight barriers to teamwork. *Personnel J*. January: 18–21.

[101]McKeen E, Billings JA. Reimbursement for physician services under the Medicare benefit. *Hospice Update*. Gainesville, Fla.: American Academy of Hospice and Palliative Medicine; December 5, 1991.

[102]Kinzbrunner BM. The role of the physician in hospice. *Hospice J*. New York: Haworth Press; 1997;12(2):49–55.

[103]Hadlock DC. Physicians' roles in hospice care. In: Corr CA, Coor DM, ed. *Hospice Care, Principles and Practice*. New York: Springer; 1983. Cited by: Kinzbrunner BM. The role of the physician in hospice. *Hospice J*. New York: Haworth Press; 1997;12(2):49–55.

[104]Johanson GA, Johanson IV. The core team. In: Sheehan DC, Forman WB, eds. *Hospice and Palliative Care: Concepts and Practice*. Boston: Jones and Bartlett; 1996:31–40.

[105]Martinez JM. The interdisciplinary team. In: Sheehan DC, Forman WB, eds. *Hospice and Palliative Care: Concepts and Practice*. Boston: Jones and Bartlett; 1996:21–29.

[106]Szczepaniak L. Additional team members. In: Sheehan DC, Forman WB, eds. *Hospice and Palliative Care: Concepts and Practice*. Boston: Jones and Bartlett; 1996:49.

[107]Cassin CJ. *Ethics of Universal Access to Palliative Care*. Presented at: Medicine at Life's End: Ethics and Humanities in Palliative Medicine. American Academy of Hospice and Palliative Medicine. March 14–15, 1997. Colorado Springs, Colo.

[108]Zerwekh J. Hospice nursing practice: what's in the literature? *Fanfare*. Hospice Nurses Association. 1996;10(3):4–5.

[109]Liaschenko J. Making a bridge: the moral work with patients we do not like. *J Palliat Care*. 1994;10(3):83–89.

[110]Vachon MLS. Emotional problems in palliative medicine: patient, family, and professional. In: Doyle D, Hanks GWC, MacDonald N, eds. *Oxford Textbook of Palliative Medicine*. New York: Oxford University Press; 1993:577–605.

[111]White WL. Managing personal and organizational stress in the care of the dying. *Hospice Education Program for Nurses*. U.S. Department of Health and Human Services. DHHS Publication No. HRA 81–27. Adapted from Vachon, MLS. Motivation and stress experienced by staff working with the terminally ill.

[112]Stedeford A. *Facing Death: Patients, Families and Professionals*. London: William Heineman Medical Books Ltd.; 1984.

[113]Quill TE, Williamson PR. Health approaches to physician stress. *Arch Intern Med*. 1990;150:1857–1861.

[114]Engel G. Need for a new medical model: a challenge for biomedicine. *Science*. 1997;196:129–134, 197. Copyright 1977 by the American Association for the Advancement of Science. Quoted in: Willamson DS, Noel ML. Systemic family medicine: an evolving concept. In: Rakel RE. *Textbook of Family Medicine*, 4th ed. Philadelphia: WB Saunders; 1990:61–79.

[115]Estés CP. *Women Who Run with the Wolves: Myths and Stories of the Wild Woman Archetype.* New York: Ballantine Books; 1992:15, 20.

[116]Bird J, Hall A, Maguire P, Heavey A. Workshops for consultants on the teaching of clinical communication skills. *Med Educ.* 1993;27(2):181–185. Cited by: Fallowfield L. Giving sad and bad news. *Lancet.* 1993;341:476–478.

[117]Maguire P, Fairbairn S, Fletcher C. Consultation skills of young doctors: I-benefits of feedback training in interviewing as students persist. *BMJ.* 1986;292:1573–1578. Cited by: Fallowfield L. Giving sad and bad news. *Lancet.* 1993;341:476–478.

[118]Bensing J. Doctor–patient communication and the quality of care. *Soc Sci Med.* 1991;32(11):1301–1310.

[119]Lichter I, Mooney J, Boyd M. Biography as therapy. *Palliat Med.* 1993;7:133–137.

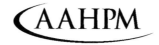

AAHPM

American Academy of Hospice and Palliative Medicine

UNIPAC Five: Caring for the Terminally Ill—Communication and the Physician's Role on the Interdisciplinary Team

Physicians are eligible to receive 6 credit hours in Category 1 of the AMA/PRA by completing and returning this posttest answer sheet to the AAHPM. Photocopies of this form will not be accepted for CME credit. The Academy will keep a record of AMA/PRA Category 1 credit hours and the record will be provided on request; however, physicians are responsible for reporting their own Category 1 CME credits when applying for the AMA/PRA or for other certificates or credentials.

Name

Street

City/State/Zip Code

Telephone

Social Security Number

Please mail this answer sheet and a check for $45.00 made out to the American Academy of Hospice and Palliative Medicine to:

Physician Training Programs
American Academy of Hospice
and Palliative Medicine
4700 W. Lake Avenue
Glenview, Illinois 60023-1485

Please circle the one correct answer for each question

1. A B C D	14. A B C D	27. A B C D
2. A B C D	15. A B C D	28. A B C D
3. A B C D	16. A B C D	29. A B C D
4. A B C D	17. A B C D	30. A B C D
5. A B C D	18. A B C D	31. A B C D
6. A B C D	19. A B C D	32. A B C D
7. A B C D	20. A B C D	33. A B C D
8. A B C D	21. A B C D	34. A B C D
9. A B C D	22. A B C D	35. A B C D
10. A B C D	23. A B C D	36. A B C D
11. A B C D	24. A B C D	37. A B C D
12. A B C D	25. A B C D	38. A B C D
13. A B C D	26. A B C D	